D1399954

Podiatric Medicine and Surgery
A Monograph series

Managing Editor: Morton D. Fielding, D.P.M.

Clinical Podiatric Laboratory Diagnosis

by

Murray J. Politz, D.P.M., F.A.C.F.S.

Fellow, American College of Foot Surgeons

Member, American Academy of Podiatric Sports Medicine

Chief of Podiatry Staff, Holy Cross Hospital,
Silver Springs, Maryland

Member Podiatry Staff, Doctors' Hospital,
Washington, D.C.

Consultant, Maryland Podiatry Residency Program

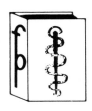

FUTURA PUBLISHING COMPANY, INC.
Mount Kisco, New York
1977

Copyright © 1977
Futura Publishing Company, Inc.

Published by
Futura Publishing Company, Inc.
295 Main Street
Mount Kisco, New York 10549

L.C. #: 77-80657
ISBN #: 0-87993-063-2

Dedication

This book is dedicated to my wife Cookie and our children, Michael, Jodi, and Brian.

Special Acknowledgments

The preparation of this book would not have been possible without the assistance of those individuals devoted to clinical laboratory work. I wish to acknowledge Dr. Sibinovic at Bionetics Research Laboratory, the staff at National Health Laboratories and special acknowledgment to Mr. Sami Sbitani of Columbia Medical Laboratories for his interest and encouragement.

I would like to especially thank my parents, Percy and Sylvia, whose many sacrifices through my years of schooling made possible this text.

The one person who deserves all the credit and accolades for everything I have accomplished professionally is my wife Cookie. I have never thanked her publicly and rarely, I am sorry to say, privately. She not only assisted in the preparation of the book, but also typed the original manuscript. She has lovingly accepted my sacrifices of time and attention belonging to her and to our children on behalf of Podiatry. Cookie, thank you.

Table of Contents

CHAPTER 1
Introduction

The purpose of this book is to serve as a review of the laboratory diagnosis of the more common ailments that affect our patients. The material presented is not original; it is, however, collated from many sources and condensed in order to give to the doctor of podiatric medicine a better understanding of the rationales involved in laboratory diagnosis. Since this book has been compiled over a long period of time, I might have inadvertently used material without acknowledging the source. This was in no manner my intent and to the best of my ability I have tried to give due and proper credit to all sources.

There are numerous types of instruments for in-office laboratory determinations which explain test procedures sufficiently. For this reason, I did not attempt to discuss reagents necessary for each test. I felt that a more medical approach to explain disease and metabolic system changes as evidenced in laboratory results was an approach that was needed. This text therefore explains disease processes with special emphasis on laboratory results.

Competent and helpful clinical laboratory directors and operators can be an invaluable source of practical advice whether you use an outside laboratory or perform the test in your office. It is best to remember that the indiscriminate multiple ordering of tests for diagnostic purposes is considered poor medical practice. The laboratory is just one diagnostic tool available to the podiatrist and should be used as such. The confirmation of diagnosis by clinical laboratory means is the most efficient use of this service. Other uses of clinical laboratory test results are in screening for occult disease, differential diagnosis determinations, ascertaining the severity of a disease, determining the stage of a disease, aiding in decisions of therapy of drug dosages, preparing for surgery or hospital admission, monitoring response during therapy, following up after completion of therapy, aiding in genetic counselling, and meeting the concerns of the medicolegal aspects of patient care.

This text is cross-referenced with normal test values, significance of tests, disease processes and screening tests. I would suggest to my readers that they give the material presented herein a thorough first reading and then that they keep the book handy in the office for speedy reference to those pathological conditions which may be diagnosed by laboratory means.

CHAPTER 2
Serologic Methods

There are four general classes of procedures used in the routine serology laboratory. They are: Agglutination, Precipitation, Complement Fixation (CF), and Fluorescent Antibody (FA). For practical purposes they measure the reaction between antibody and antigen. These serologic tests are used in the diagnosis of syphilis, salmonella, brucella, tularemia, streptococcal infections, hepatitis, thyroid diseases, collagen and parasitic diseases.

Since it is important for podiatrists to understand antibody and antigen reactions, the following examples and explanations may be helpful.

ANTIGEN

An antigen is any substance which, when introduced into an individual who lacks that substance, stimulates the production of an antibody and which, when mixed with the specific antibody, reacts with it in some observable way such as agglutination, hemolysis, or precipitation.

ANTIBODY

An antibody is a specific substance produced by an individual in response to the introduction of an antigen.

ANTISTREPTOCOCCAL ANTIBODIES

The serologic response to group A streptococcal infections has been extensively used because the documentation by culture methods is often lacking in patients suspected of having acute glomerulonephritis or acute rheumatic fever. The antibodies most often used in clinical situations are antistreptolysin-O (ASO), antihyaluronidase (AH), antistreptokinase, antidesoxyribonuclease B (anti DNA-B), and antidiphosphopyridine nucleotidase (anti DPN-ase).

3

Group A streptococcal infections are most common in school-age children; however, antistreptococcal antibodies are found in significant levels in healthy individuals. The ASO is the most important serologic procedure in patients with suspected nonsuppurative sequelae of streptococcal infections. It is important to remember that children under two years of ago have ASO titres of less than 50 units because streptococcal infections are rare in this age group. Children five to twelve years are repeatedly exposed to streptococcus and will often have an ASO titre up to 200 units. In adults the range is about 125 units. The antidesoxyribonuclease (anti-DNASE-B) antibody is especially useful in patients with streptococcal pyoderma.

AUTOANTIBODIES

The testing for autoantibodies may be performed using the direct antiglobulin (Coomb's) test for antibodies attached to red cells and the indirect antiglobulin (Coomb's test ICT) which detects free autoantibodies in the serum.

THE COOMB'S TEST

The Coomb's test demonstrates autoimmune antibodies which are incomplete antibodies. They are antibodies which are absorbed on the surface of red cells and are incomplete in the sense that they do not cause agglutination or hemolysis when the cells are mixed with saline dilutions of the patient's own serum.

The direct Coomb's test is best performed in a quantitative manner with different concentrations of antiglobulin serum. A positive result from a direct Coomb's test demonstrated the presence of autoimmune antibodies and suggests hemolytic anemia. A false positive result from a direct Coomb's test demonstrates the presence of auto-rheumatoid arthritis, leukemia, and aplastic anemia.

The indirect Coomb's test is used to detect 1) the presence of free auto-antibodies in the serum of patients with acquired hemolytic anemia and 2) RH antibodies in the sera of antenatal patients.

AUTOIMMUNE DISEASES

Autoimmune diseases are diseases in which the antigen is an autoantigen and the antibody is an autoantibody. Idiopathic and symptomatic autoimmune hemolytic anemia, autoimmune leuko-penia, and paroxysmal cold hemoglobinuria are examples.

COMPLEMENT FIXATION TEST

Complement Fixation tests are antigen-antibody interactions which form the basis for laboratory tests used in the identification of antigens and antibodies involved in disease processes.

COLD AGGLUTININS

Cold agglutinins or cold-reacting antibodies are antibodies for type O erythrocytes at 0° to 10°C and may be found in such acute infections as mycoplasma pneumonia, infectious mononucleosis, trypanosomiasis, and congenital cytomegalovirus infection.

C-REACTIVE PROTEIN (CRP)

The C-reactive protein is classified as an acute phase reactant that has been found in patients with a wide variety of infectious diseases caused by both gram positive and gram negative bacteria and non-infectious inflammatory conditions. The elevation of CRP is non-specific and is only an indicator of acute response which is similar to the Erythrocyte Sedimentation Rate (ESR). It rises faster and returns to normal faster than the ESR, usually in 8−10 days.

The CRP may be elevated in bacterial infections, in some tumors, and in various types of tissue destruction such as myocardial infarction. It is most often used to monitor patients with acute rheumatic fever and rheumatoid arthritis. It rises during the acute phase and returns to normal with appropriate therapy. Viral diseases are not associated with CRP.

The CRP is elevated in pregnancy and in patients on oral contraceptive preparations, and even in those with an IUD in place.

HEMAGGLUTINOGENS AND HEMAGGLUTININS

Antigens present on the surface of erythrocytes are referred to as hemagglutinogens and antibodies that agglutinate erythrocytes are referred to as hemagglutinins.

HETEROPHILE

Heterophile antibody titres may increase to 224 or greater in infectious mononucleosis (Figure 2-1). They also may be found in low titre in normal individuals and have been observed in serum sickness. The three heterophile antibodies may be differentiated by the laboratory by absorption with guinea pig extract.

HETEROIMMUNE DISEASES

Heteroimmune diseases are those in which the antigen is a microorganism invading the host. The antibody is produced by the host. Acute acquired hemolytic anemia in virus pneumonia and infectious mononucleosis are examples.

IMMUNOHEMATOLOGY

Immunohematology is the study of diseases of blood in which the cause or clinical manifestation has been shown to be determined by an antigen-antibody reaction.

ISOIMMUNE DISEASES

Isoimmune diseases are due to isoantibodies which are antibodies directed against an antigen foreign to the host but present in other individuals of the same species. Autoantibodies are antibodies produced by an organism against antigens present in its own cells or tissue. Transfusion reaction is a good example.

ISOIMMUNIZATION

Isoimmunization is the formation of immune antibodies by a member of a given species against some antigen normally absent from his own body but present in another member of the same species. RH positive blood transfused to a RH negative person can result in isoimmunization to the RH isoagglutinogen.

RHEUMATOID FACTOR

The rheumatoid factor is an immunoglobulin found in the serum of the rheumatoid arthritis and systemic lupus erythematosus patient, although trauma, fatigue, and emotional factors may also be etiologic in nature. The rheumatoid factor agglutinates with a number of

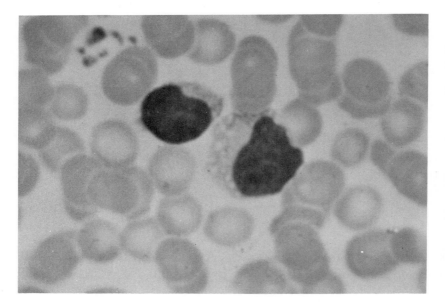

FIGURE 2-1: Atypical lymphocyte in infectious mononucleosis. (From the Armed Forces Institute of Pathology, Washington, D.C., Negative No. L-12967-21, with permission.)

suspended particles including hemolytic streptococci, sheep red blood cells sensitized with antisheep erythrocyte rabbit serum, latex, and bentonite suspensions.

SEROLOGY IN SYPHILIS

The most common tool for the diagnosis of this disease is serology. Syphilis is seldom diagnosed by demonstrating the organisms in a primary or secondary lesion. Two general groups of procedures are used: first, nontreponemal antigen tests such as the VDRL; second, the treponemal antigen test with the fluorescent treponema antibody absorbed (FTA-ABS) as an example.

The VDRL is a good test in primary and secondary syphilis but is less sensitive in the late stages. If clinical findings indicate syphilis then the FTA-ABS is indicated. The VDRL also may give a false positive result (between 10—30 percent) in which case a follow-up with a FTA-ABS should be done. This may also be positive. A false positive may be associated with pneumonia, tuberculosis, subacute bacterial endocarditis, chickenpox, infectious mononucleosis, scarlet fever, leprosy, and drug addiction; with the last two occurring most often.

SEROLOGY TABLE OF NORMAL VALUES°

Test	Normal Value
Antibovine Milk Antibodies	Negative
Antidesoxyribonuclease (ADNAase)	< 1:20
Antinuclear Antibodies (ANA)	< 1:10
Antistreptococcal Hyaluronidase (ASH)	< 1:256
Antistreptolysin O (ASL O)	< 160 Todd units
Coccidioidomycosis Antibodies	Negative
Cold Agglutinins	< 1:32
C-reactive Protein (CRP)	0
Fluorescent Treponemal Antibodies (FTA)	Non-reactive
Heterophile Antibodies	< 1:56
Latex Fixation	Negative
Leptospira Agglutinins	Negative
Rheumatoid Factor	
Sensitized sheep cell	< 1:160
Latex fixation	< 1:80
Bentonite particles	1:32
Thyroid Antibodies	
Antithyroglobulin	1:32
Antithyroid microsomal	1:56
Tularemia Agglutinins and Typhoid Agglutinins	1:80
VDRL	Non-reactive
Weil-Felix (Proteus OX-2, OX-K, OX-15 Agglutinins)	Four-fold rise in titre between acute and convalescence sera

°From Davidshohn, I. and Henry, J.B. (Eds.): *Todd-Sanford Clinical Diagnosis by Laboratory Methods*, 15th edition, W.B. Saunders Co., Philadelphia, 1974, p. 1391, with permission.

CHAPTER 3
Laboratory Tests

BLOOD°

Test Name	Specimen Required	Container Code	Normals
Acetone, semi-quant (blood)	5 ml blood or 2 ml serum	Red	Negative
Acid phosphatase	2 ml serum FROZEN°° (50% loss activity at 5 hrs. room temp.)	Red	0.04-0.70 m moles/l (Bessey-Lowery)
Albumin	5 ml blood or 2 ml serum	Red	Human: 3.5-5.0 gm/dl
Aldolase	5 ml blood or 2 ml serum	Red	1.0-6.0 mU/ml
Alkaline phosphatase	5 ml blood or 2 ml serum	Red	Human: to 1 year—63-315 mU/ml 1-12—39-290 mU/ml 13-16—30-231 mU/ml 17-99—30-105 mU/ml
Ammonia (plasma)	5 ml oxalated blood CENTRIFUGE AND SEPARATE FREEZE IMMEDIATELY	Black	$0-90 \mu g/dl$
Amylase (serum)	5 ml blood or 2 ml serum	Red	Human: 60-160 units
Anti-nuclear antibody screen	2 ml serum	Red	Reactivity: negative Patterns: not present
Bilirubin, total	5 ml blood or 2 ml serum	Red	Human: 0.2 to 1.0 mg/dl
Bilirubin, total, direct and indirect	10 ml blood or 2 ml serum	Red	Total: 0.2 to 1.0 mg/dl Direct: 0.1 to 0.5 mg/dl Indirect: 0.1 to 0.5 mg/dl

°From Bionetics Research Laboratories, Kensington, Maryland, with permission.
°°Samples that require freezing must be frozen in dry ice and methanol or in liquid nitrogen.

BLOOD (Continued)

Test Name	Specimen Required	Container Code	Normals
Bleeding time	Contact laboratory for appointment	—	3.0-7.0 mins.
Blood cell parasites	2 non-fixed blood smears	Slides	No parasites found
Blood count, automated RBC, WBC, HgB, HCT, MCV, MCH, MCHC	5 ml whole blood	Lavender	See individual components
Blood culture	10 ml whole blood or 2 ml whole blood	Broth Bottle Broth tube	No growth
Blood Indices	5 ml whole blood or	Lavender	MCV 80.0-94.0 Cuu MCH 27.0-34.0 PG MCHC 32.0-36.0%
Blood urea nitrogen (BUN)	5 ml whole blood or 3 ml serum	Red	Human: 9-24 mg/dl
Bromsulphalein (BSP)	5 ml blood or 2 ml serum, timed sample	Red	Retention: 0-5% at 45 mins. 0.2% at 60 mins.
Brucella agglutination *abortus, suis, melitensis*	2 ml serum	Red	Negative to 1:80 dilution
Calcium unbound and total	10 ml blood or 4 ml serum	Red	Total: 8.5 to 10.5 mg/dl Unbound: 50-58% of total
Carbon dioxide (bicarbonate serum)	5 ml blood or 2 ml serum	Red	Human: 24-32 MEq/l
Cephalin-cholesterol flocculation	5 ml blood or 2 ml serum	Red	Negative at 24 hrs. +1 at 48 hrs.
Chloride (serum)	5 ml blood or 2 ml serum	Red	Human: 95-105 MEq/l

BLOOD (Continued)

Test Name	Specimen Required	Container Code	Normals

Cholesterol	5 ml blood
	2 ml serum
		Red	To age 30 years:
			  120-150 mg/dl
			30 to 40 yrs:
			  130-290 mg/dl
			40 to 99 yrs:
			  150-300 mg/dl

Cholesterol esters	5 ml blood 2 ml serum	Red	105-200 mg/dl
Clot retraction	10 ml whole blood	Blue	Over 65% in 24 hrs.
Coagulation (Lee White)	Contact laboratory for appointment		7.0-15.0 mins.
Coccidiomy-cosis (screen)	2 ml serum	Red	Negative
Cold agglutinins	2 ml serum, *Keep at 37° temperature before separating*	Red	Negative
Coomb's test, direct	5 ml blood	Red	Negative
Coomb's test, indirect	5 ml blood or 2 ml serum	Red	Negative
Cortiocosteroids (plasma)	10 ml blood or 4 ml plasma	Green	5-25 μg/dl
Creatine (serum)	10 ml blood or 4 ml serum	Red	Male: 0.17-0.50 mg/dl Female: 0.35-0.93 mg/dl
Creatine phos-phokinase (CPK)	5 ml blood or 2 ml serum	Red	Male: 40-130 μIU/ml Female: 40-120 μIU/ml
Creatinine (serum)	5 ml blood or 2 ml serum	Red	0.7-1.4 mg/dl
Creatinine clearance	2 ml serum + 100 ml timed urine speci-men, record total volume	Red, White	Clearance = 90-120 ml/min.

BLOOD (Continued)

Test Name	Specimen Required	Container Code	Normals
C-reactive protein	2 ml serum	Red	2 hour—negative 24 hour—negative
Cryoglobulins, qual.	5 ml blood, *DO NOT REFRIGERATE*	Red	Negative
Crystal identification (synovial fluid)	1.0 ml synovial fluid	Red	Negative for crystals
Culture (blood)	10 ml blood in vacutainer bottle with media or 2 ml blood in vacutainer tube with media	Sterile container	No organisms isolated
Factor II (prothrombin assay)	1 ml plasma, *FROZEN*, contact laboratory before drawing specimen	Blue	Over 85% of control
Factor VIII	1 ml plasma, *FROZEN*, contact laboratory before drawing specimen	Blue	Over 85% of control
Factor aaIX	1 ml plasma, *FROZEN*, contact laboratory before drawing specimen	Blue	Over 85% of control
Factor X	1 ml plasma, *FROZEN*, contact laboratory before drawing specimen	Blue	Over 85% of control
Factor XI	1 ml plasma, *FROZEN*, contact laboratory before drawing specimen	Blue	Over 85% of control
Febrile Agglut. and antigen	2 ml serum	Red	Negative at 1:80 dilution for each antigen tested
Typhoid O	2 ml serum	Red	Negative at 1:80 dilution for each antigen tested

BLOOD (Continued)

Test Name	Specimen Required	Container Code	Normals
Typhoid H	2 ml serum	Red	Negative at 1:80 dilution for each antigen tested
Paratyphoid A	2 ml serum	Red	Negative at 1:80 dilution for each antigen tested
Paratyphoid B	2 ml serum	Red	Negative at 1:80 dilution for each antigen tested
Brucella abortus	2 ml serum	Red	Negative at 1:80 dilution for each antigen tested
Proteus OXK	2 ml serum	Red	Negative at 1:80 dilution for each antigen tested
Proteus OX19	2 ml serum	Red	Negative at 1:80 dilution for each antigen tested
Proteus OX2	2 ml serum	Red	Negative at 1:80 dilution for each antigen tested
Fibrinogen	5 ml whole blood	Black or Blue	200-450 mg/dl
Fluorescent treponemal	2 ml serum	Red	Non-reactive
Globulin, protein	5 ml blood or 2 ml serum	Red	2.2-3.8 mg/dl
Glucose (fasting)	3 ml blood or 2 ml plasma	Grey	60-120 mg/dl
Glucose, 2-hr. post-prandial (blood)	3 ml whole blood or 1 ml plasma	Grey	60-120 mg/dl
Glucose tolerance (6-hr.)	3 ml whole blood per tube or 1 ml plasma per tube, 10 ml urine (optional)	Grey White	Fasting: 60-120 mg/dl ½ hour—95-165 mg/dl 1 hour—95-165 mg/dl 2 hour—60-120 mg/dl 3 hour—60-120 mg/dl 4 hour—65-120 mg/dl 5 hour—65-120 mg/dl 6 hour—65-120 mg/dl Urines negative
Hemotocrit (PVC) packed cell volume	5 ml whole blood	Lavender	Male: 42-52 Vol % Female: 37-47 Vol %

BLOOD (Continued)

Test Name	Specimen Required	Container Code	Normals
Hemoglobin (HgB)	5 ml whole blood	Lavender	Male: 14-18 gm % Female: 12-16 gm %
Hepatitis-associated antigen (RIA)(HAA)	2 ml serum	Red	Negative
17-hydroxycor-ticosteroids (serum)	20 ml blood or 10 ml serum	Red	5-20 mg/ml
Iron binding capacity	10 ml blood or 3 ml serum	Red	250-350 μg/dl
17-ketosteroids, total (serum)	10 ml serum, *SEPARATE FROM CELLS IMMEDIATELY*	Red	Male: 40-130 μg/dl Female: 25-100 μg/dl
Lactic dehydro-genase (LDH)	2 ml serum	Red	100-225 mU/ml
Lipase (serum)	10 ml blood or 3 ml serum	Red	0-1.0 units/ml
Lipid, total (serum)	5 ml blood or 2 ml serum	Red	400-1000 mg/dl
Lupus erythe-matosus (LE)	10 ml clotted blood	Red	No LE cells seen
Methemo-globin	3 ml whole blood *(SAMPLE FROZEN)*	Green	0-0.25 mg/dl 0.4-1.5% of total Hgb
Mononucleo-sis screen	2 ml serum	Red	Negative
Neisseria gonorrhea C.F. test	2 ml serum	Red	Negative
Partial throm-boplastin time (PTT) non-activated	Contact laboratory	Blue	40.0-100.0

BLOOD (Continued)

Test Name	Specimen Required	Container Code	Normals
Phenolsulfon-phthalein (PSP)	Entire urine specimens collected at 15-30-60 and 120 min. intervals, and labeled, contact laboratory for instructions	White	15 mins.: 20-50% 30 mins.: 16-24% 60 mins.: 9-17% 120 mins.: 3-10%
Phosphorus (serum)	2 ml serum	Red	2.5-4.5 mg/dl
Platelet count	5 ml whole blood	Lavender	200-400 K/cumm
Potassium (serum)	2 ml serum; *SEPARATE SERUM WITHIN ONE HOUR*	Red	3.5-5.0 MEq/1
Protein, total, albumin, globulin, A/G ratio	5 ml blood or 2 ml serum	Red	Total protein: 6.0-8.0 gm/dl Albumin: 3.5-5.0 gm/dl Globulin: 2.2-3.8 gm/dl A/G ratio: 1.1-1.9 gm/dl
Protein electro phoresis (serum), total protein albumin, A-1 globulin, A-2 globulin, B-globulin, Y-globulin, A/G ratio	5 ml blood or 2 ml serum	Red	Total protein: 6.0-8.0 gm/dl Albumin: 47-70% Alpha, globulin: 2.7-5.8% Alpha$_2$ globulin: 5.1-12.0% Beta globulin: 4.5-15.7% Gamma globulin: 11.3-24.0% A/G ratio: 1.1-1.9
Protein, total (serum)	5 ml blood or 2 ml serum	Red	6.0-8.0 gm/dl
Prothrombin time	5 ml whole blood (oxalated)	Black	Over 85% of control
Rheumatoid arthritis (RA) latex slide screen	2 ml serum	Red	Negative

BLOOD (Continued)

Test Name	Specimen Required	Container Code	Normals
Reticulocyte count	5 ml whole blood	Lavender	0.5-1.5%
Schilling differential:	Blood smear	*SLIDE*	
Bands			0-3 percent
Seg. neutophilis			51-67 percent
Lymphocytes			25-33 percent
Monocytes			2-6 percent
Eosinophils			1-4 percent
Basophils			0-1 percent
Platelets			Adequate
Atypical lymphs			None
Anisocytosis			None
Hypochromia			None
Poikilocytosis			None
NRBC			None
Sedimentation rate (ESR) (Westergren)	5 ml whole blood	Lavender	Male: 0-9.0 mm/hr Female: 0-20.0 mm/hr
Sedimentation rate (Wintrobe)	5 ml whole blood	Lavender	ESR CSR (Male): 0-9.0 mm/hr CRS (Female): 0-20.0 mm/hr
SGOT (glutamic oxalacetic transaminase)	5 ml blood or 2 ml serum, *REFRIGERATE*	Red	10-40 mU/ml
SGPT (glutamic pyruvic transaminase)	5 ml blood or 2 ml serum, *REFRIGERATE*	Red	5-30 mU/ml
Sickle-cell screen	5 ml whole blood	Lavender	Negative
Sodium (serum)	2 ml serum	Red	135-145 MEq/1
Testosterone (blood-RIA)	20 ml blood or 10 ml serum	Red	Male: $3.00-8.00\mu g/ml$ Female: $.25-1.00\mu g/ml$

BLOOD (Continued)

Test Name	Specimen Required	Container Code	Normals
Thromboplastin generation	1 ml plasma + 1 ml serum, *FROZEN*	Blue + Red	7-16 secs.
Thyrobinding index (TBI)	5 ml blood or 2 ml serum	Red	0.9-1.1
Thyroxine (t4), RIA T₃ uptake, calculated T₇	10 ml blood or 2 ml serum	Red	3.9-14.7 μg/dl
Triglycerides	5 ml blood or 2 ml serum, *FASTING*	Red	Humans: 0-29 yrs: 10-140 mg/dl 30-39 yrs: 10-150 mg/dl 40-49 yrs: 10-160 mg/dl 50-59 yrs: 10-190 mg/dl
Uric acid (serum)	3 ml serum	Red	Male: 2.5-8.0 mg/dl Female: 1.5-6.5 mg/dl
VDRL, qual., if positive do VDRL, quant. and FTA	3 ml serum	Red	VDRL-nonreactive, no titer FTA-nonreactive
Viral serology (HAI)	10 ml blood or 3 ml serum from acute and convalescent stages (specify virus from list)	2 Red	Negative for selected virus
Vitamin A (Retinol)	10 ml blood or 3 ml serum, *DO NOT EXPOSE TO LIGHT, WRAP IN FOIL*	Red	Adult: 20-80 mg/dl Infant: 10-60 mg/dl

URINE*

Test Name	Specimen Required	Container Code	Normals
Acetone, semi-quant. (urine)	5 ml urine	Blue	Negative
Addis count	12-hr urine, entire amount, record total volume, rinse container with formalin	C	RBC: 0-0.5 M/12 hrs. WBC: 0-1.0 M/12 hrs. Epithelial cells: 0-0.8 m/12 hrs. Casts: 0-5 K/12 hrs.
Amylase (urine)	2-hr timed urine sample or 250 ml aliquot (note time period covered and total volume)	White	0-300 units/hr.
Bence-Jones protein, qual.	10 ml urine	Plastic container no preservative	Negative
Bilirubin, qual. (urine)	10 ml urine	White	Negative
Calcium, quant. (urine)	24-hr urine or 250 mg aliquot + 15 ml HCl, record total volume	Special	50-150 mg/24 hrs.
Calcium, qual. (Sulkowitch)	5 ml urine	Blue	Negative
Catecholamines	24-hr urine or 250 ml aliquot, acidified during collection to pH 1-2 by adding 15 ml concentrated HCl	Special	0-115 μg/24 hrs.
Chloride (urine)	24-hr urine or 250 ml aliquot, record total volume	White	110-250 MEq/24 hrs.

*From Bionetics Research Laboratories, Kensington, Maryland, with permission.

URINE (Continued)

Test Name	Specimen Required	Container Code	Normals
Creatine (urine)	24-hr urine or 100 ml aliquot, record total volume	White	Male: 0-40 mg/24 hrs. Female: 0-80 mg/24 hrs.
Creatinine	24-hr urine or 100 ml aliquot, record total volume	White	0.8-1.9 gm/24 hrs.
Glucose, quant.	100 ml of 24 hrs. urine, record total volume	White with 10 mg NaF	0-0.1 gm/dl
Glucose, semi-quant.	5 ml urine	Blue	Negative
17-hydroxy-corticoster-oids—total (ketogenic)	24-hr. urine or 250 ml aliquot, record total volume	C	Male: 5-23 mg/24 hrs. Female: 3-15 mg/24 hrs.
17-ketosteroids, total	24-hr. urine or 250 ml aliquot, record total volume	C	Male: 9-22 mg/24 hrs. Female: 6-15 mg/24 hrs.
Melanin, qual.	50 ml urine	White	Negative
Occult blood	5 ml urine	Blue	Negative
Phosphorous	24-hr urine or 250 ml aliquot, record total volume	White	0.9-1.3 gm/24 hrs.
pH reaction	5 ml urine	Blue	5.0-9.0 pH units
Porphyrins, qual.	30 ml urine add 5 gm sodium carbonate, *MUST NOT BE EXPOSED TO LIGHT OR PUT IN CONTACT WITH METAL*	White	Negative
Potassium	24-hr urine or 250 ml aliquot, record total volume	White	25-100 MEq/24 hrs.

URINE (Continued)

Test Name	Specimen Required	Container Code	Normals
Protein electro-phoresis (urine), total protein albumin, A-1 globulin, A-2 globulin, B-globulin, Y-globulin, A/G ratio	250 ml aliquot urine or 24-hr collection, record total volume	Blue	Total protein: 10-100 mg/24 hrs. Albumin: 35-46 Alpha globulin: 25-30 Alpha$_2$ globulin: 15-20 Beta globulin: 5-10 Gamma globulin: 3-10 A/G ratio: 0.38-0.61
Protein, semi-quant.	5 ml urine	Blue	Negative
Protein, total, quant.	250 ml aliquot or total 24-hr collection record total volume	Blue	10-100 mg/24 hrs.
Sodium	250 ml aliquot or total 24-hr collection record total volume	C	130-260 MEq/24 hrs.
Specific gravity	15 ml urine	White	1.001-1.035
Urea clearance	Two timed urine samples and total volumes recorded + 1-5 ml blood	2 White + Red Height weight, and age	Narrative
Uric acid	24-hr urine or 250 aliquot, record total volume	C	250-750 mg/24 hrs.

URINE (Continued)

Test Name	Specimen Required	Container Code	Normals
Urinalysis (microscopic)	25 ml urine	Blue	WBC—0-10/hpf RBC—0-4/hpf Casts—0/hpf Epithelial cells—0-10/hpf Amorphous sediment—1-4+ Bacteria—negative Mucous threads—1-4+ Crystals present—name Other—identify
Urobilinogen, qual.	Random urine	White	Negative
Vanillylmandelic acid (VMA)	24-hr urine or 250 ml aliquot	Special acidified with 15 ml HCl	0-10 mg/24 hrs.

CHAPTER 4
Hematology

BLOOD CONSTITUENTS

The blood consists of fluid called plasma in which are suspended erythrocytes, leukocytes, and platelets. When blood coagulates, the fluid that remains after the clot is removed is called serum. Serum differs from plasma by the loss of protein fibrinogen. The two sources of blood for laboratory tests are capillary (peripheral) or venous blood. For most examinations venous blood is preferred; however, there are times when a differential count or follow-up hemoglobin or hematocrit may be taken from the lobe of an ear, the palmar surface of a finger, or, in infants, from the plantar surface of the great toe or heel.

VENIPUNCTURE

With the exception of glucose, triglycerides, and inorganic phosphorus most blood chemical constituents reveal no significant change after a standard meal. Therefore, it is not essential for a patient to be in an absolute fasting state prior to blood specimen collection. It is always wise to remember that some patients do faint when a blood sample is taken. They should be lying down or seated with their feet elevated and the back of the chair slightly reclined. The arm should hang down so that gravity will fill the veins in the arm. The arm can then be rested on the arm chair and the tourniquet applied above the elbow. The rubber tourniquet should be applied so that the last turn is tucked in in such a manner that a slight pull on the end will release it. The patient should then open and close his fist and the veins should be prominent. If veins are not prominent they can usually be felt beneath the skin with the index finger.

The skin is then swabbed with a pad of 70% alcohol and allowed to dry. The vein is fixed into position by stretching the skin, proximal to the puncture site with the thumb. The syringe or Vacutainer®° holder is held between the thumb and the last three fingers of the other hand. The index finger rests against the hub of the needle and

°Becton-Dickinson & Co., Rutherford, New Jersey

23

acts as a guide. The opening at the end of the needle should point up-wards and the vein can be entered with a quick direct puncture of both skin and vein.

After the samples have been taken the patient may release the fist and the tourniquet is released. A sterile gauze pad is placed with firm pressure as the opposite hand removes the needle. The patient may then apply firm pressure on the pad and elevate the arm for a few minutes to stop bleeding and prevent hematoma. After all bleeding has stopped the arm may be swabbed or sprayed with an antiseptic and a small Band-aid®° applied.

Venipuncture with a Vacutainer®°° system has largely replaced sample collection with a syringe and needle; however, when poor veins are encountered I recommend a 10–20 cc syringe with a 20 G one-inch needle. The syringe is then emptied into the Vacutainer® system. This system provides flexibility in terms of volume (2, 3, 5, 7, or 20 ml per tube) and anticoagulant (heparin, oxalate, citrate or ethylenediaminetriacetic acid salts [EDTA]), and sterile tubes. An adapter is available with the holder for different gauge needles. The rubber stoppers are color coded to distinguish whether the test tube contains a certain anticoagulant, is plain, or is a special tube (see Figure 4-1).

The disposable needle screws into the holder and the tube is placed in the holder so that the rubber stopper is slightly imbedded into the short needle inside the rubber stopper. After the needle is in-serted into the vein the holder is stabilized with one hand and the tube is pushed all the way into the holder. The vacuum is thus broken and the blood flows into the tube. If another tube is needed, the original tube is removed after it is full and another tube is inserted all the way into the holder. After samples have been taken, the whole unit is withdrawn.

Corning has introduced a new red top vacuum tube called the Corvac®† tube. The tube is allowed to fill with blood, inverted, al-lowed to clot for thirty minutes, centrifuged for fifteen minutes, and sent to the laboratory in a normal manner with the serum separated if it is to be mailed. From this sample of blood most chemical blood tests can be run without the need of several different type tubes.

PUNCTURE FOR CAPILLARY BLOOD

The technique of puncture should first include cleaning the site

°Johnson & Johnson, New Brunswick, New Jersey
°°Becton-Dickinson & Co., Rutherford, New Jersey
†Dow Corning, Midlands, Michigan

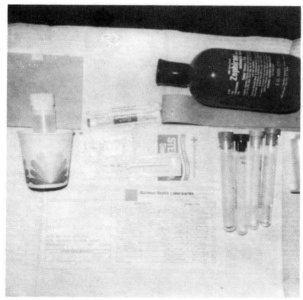

FIGURE 4-1: Routine blood and urine collection set up in office. Note Vacutainer® system with several tubes.

with a pad of 70% alcohol and rubbing to increase the amount of blood in the part. When the skin has dried a puncture of 2—3 mm in depth is made with a disposable blade or lancet. A deliberate quick firm stab wound is made deep and the first drop of blood is wiped away because it contains tissue juices. The blood should not be pressed or squeezed out since this will dilute the specimen with fluid from the tissue. The blood is drawn by either a capillary tube or a pipette. After the sample is taken a dry sterile dressing is held on the part with slight pressure until bleeding subsides.

TECHNIQUE OF BLOOD SLIDES

The blood is obtained as outlined in the sample blood collection. A small drop of blood is placed almost to one end of a slide. The slide is placed on a flat surface. With the thumb and forefinger of the right hand, hold the end of a second slide against the surface of the first at an angle of 30 to 40 degrees and draw it back against the drop of blood until contact is established. The drop will run across the end of the slide on contact. Pushing the top slide forward so that the blood spreads evenly on the bottom slide is done with moderate speed using only the weight of the top slide. Contact should remain until all the blood has been spread in a thin film.

The slide should be made evenly and quickly and dried fast so that a true clinical picture can be determined (see Figure 4-2).

MICROSCOPIC EXAMINATION

For microscopic examination of blood the polychromatic stain or Wright's stain is most often used. The varying colors help distinguish the different cells. This is the best means to study morphology. The red cells are pink, the nuclei of leukocytes are purplish blue, the eosinophilic granules are red-orange, the basophil has dark bluish purple granules, the platelets have dark lilac granules, and the cytoplasm of lymphlocytes is robin-egg blue.

ERYTHROCYTES

In normal slides they appear as circular, homogenous discs of uniform size from 6–8 μm in diameter. The center is slightly paler than the periphery.

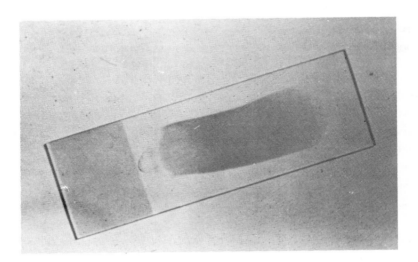

FIGURE 4-2: Thin blood film stained with Wright's (eosin azure methylene blue) stain.

PATHOLOGY

The depth of staining gives a rough guide to the amount of hemoglobin in red cells. Normochromic refers to the normal intensity of staining. When the amount of hemoglobin is decreased the central area becomes paler and larger and the condition is termed hypochromic. The MCH and MCHC are usually decreased. Red cells which are larger and thicker stain deeper with less central pallor, as in megaloblastic anemia and are hyperchromic. They have an increased MCH but the MCHC is normal. The presence of a slide which has hypochromic cells and normochromic cells is termed anisochromic or dimorphic anemia.

The size of cells is important to note: microcytosis (small), macrocytosis (large), and anisocytosis (different sizes). The size of the cells should mean cell volume not diameter (Figure 4-3).

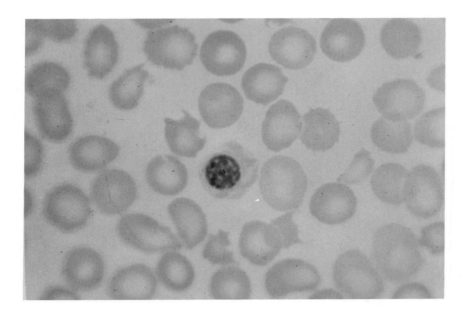

FIGURE 4-3: A marked variation in shape (poikilocytosis) and size (anisocytosis) of red cells in hemolytic anemia. Note rubrocyte in center. (From the Armed Forces Institute of Pathology, Washington, D.C., Negative No. L-12967-64, with permission.)

Variation in the shape of the cell is called poikilocytosis. There are several types of poikilocytes that are seen in different disease processes. Elliptocytes are elliptically shaped cells seen in hereditary elliptocytosis, iron-deficiency anemia, myelofibrosis, myeloid metaplasia, megaloblastic anemias, and sickle-cell anemia. Spherocytes are spherical-shaped erythrocytes found in hereditary spherocytosis, in some acquired hemolytic anemias, and where there has been direct physical or chemical injury to the cells as in body burns. Target cells are thinner and show a peripheral rim of hemoglobin with a dark central hemoglobin area. These areas are separated by a pale unstained ring containing less hemoglobin. They may be seen in obstructive jaundice post-splenectomy, and any hypochromic anemia such as thalassemia, and hemoglobin C disease. Schistocytes are cell fragments which indicate hemolysis as found in megaloblastic anemia, in severe burns, or in microangiopathic hemolytic anemia (Figure 4-4).

Variations in structure also occur in pathologic states. Basophilic stippling with basophilic granules in the erythrocytes may be seen in

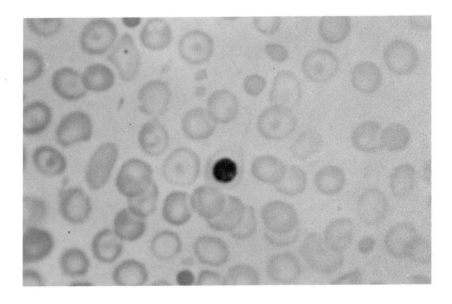

FIGURE 4-4: Target cells, spherocytes, small fragments of red cells (schizocytes) and a nucleated red cell. (From the Armed Forces Institute of Pathology, Washington, D.C., Negative No. L-12967-7, with permission.)

increased production of red cells, lead poisoning, severe anemia, or other diseases of impaired hemoglobin synthesis (Figure 4-5). Howell-Jolly Bodies are round particles of nuclear chromatin which may be seen in the red blood cell in megaloblastic anemia, hemolytic anemia, and post-splenectomy (Figure 4-6). Cabot Rings are loop-shaped structures occasionally seen in pernicious anemia, lead poisoning and other erythropoietic disorders (Figure 4-7).

RETICULOCYTE COUNT

The reticulocyte count and evaluation is perhaps the simplest measure of effective erythropoiesis. RNA is present for a day or two after the entrance of the very young erythrocyte and staining of the cell results in a diffuse basophilia. The normal absolute reticulocyte count is approximately 50,000 per microliter or one percent of the circulating erythrocytes. An increase may be interpreted as indicating both an excessive demand for new erythrocytes and a competent mar-

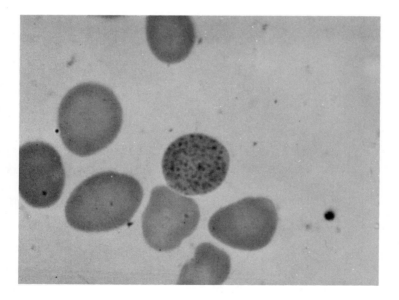

FIGURE 4-5: Basophilic stippling of red cells in hemolytic anemia. (From the Armed Forces Institute of Pathology, Washington, D.C., Negative No. L-12967-39, with permission.)

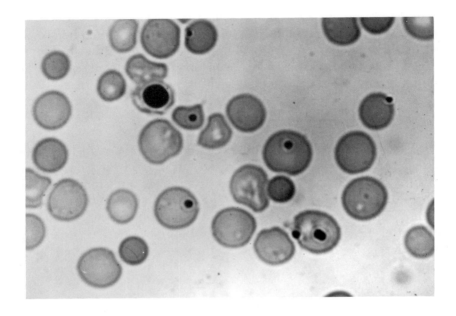

FIGURE 4-6: Howell-Jolly bodies in hemolytic anemia with thromocytopenia. The majority of red cells containing these nucleus fragments are macrocytic in addition to varying in size (anisocytosis) and in shape (poikilocytosis). The small, deeply stained red cells are spherocytes. (From the Armed Forces Institute of Pathology, Washington, D.C., Negative No. L-12967-108, with permission.)

row. A decrease may be due to failure in bone marrow function or a disease demand of the body. A normal individual with a normal supply of iron can increase red cell production by 2—3 times normal within a week of the hematocrit decrease.

HEMOGLOBIN

Hemoglobin, the main component of the red cells, is a conjugated protein that carries oxygen and carbon dioxide. Concentration of hemoglobin is expressed in grams per 100 ml of blood. Methods used in measurement of the concentration of hemoglobin in the blood, or hemoglobinometry, can be divided into four main classes: colorimetric, gasometric, specific gravity, and chemical.

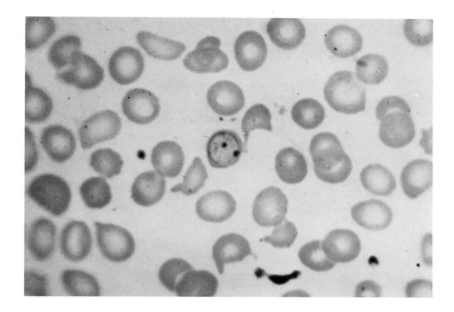

FIGURE 4-7: An erythrocyte with a Cabot Ring, two Howell-Jolly bodies and basophilic stippling seen in a patient with chronic granulocytic leukemia. (From the Armed Forces Institute of Pathology, Washington, D.C., Negative No. L-12967-68, with permission.)

HEMATOCRIT

The hematocrit in a sample is the volume of erythrocytes expressed as a percentage of the volume of whole blood. The hematocrit reflects the concentration of red cells, not the total red-cell mass. A low hematocrit indicates anemia, and a high hematocrit indicates polycythemia. The hematocrit is measured by either the macromethod of Wintrobe or by the micromethod utilizing a small capillary tube which is sealed and centrifuged (Figure 4-8).

BLOOD CELL COUNTING

Blood cell counting, that is, the number of specific cells in a specific volume, is seldom done manually except for platelet counts.

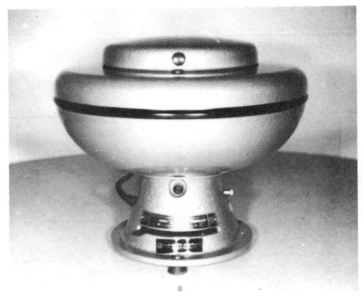

FIGURE 4-8: Clinical tabletop centrifuge.

Red and white cell counting pipettes and chambers with diluting fluid were utilized in the past; they are now largely replaced by electronic counters. Electronic counters are either based on changes in electrical resistance by the cells which are counted as voltage pulses or by deflection in a light beam by cells which are converted to electric pulses by a photomultiplier tube (Figure 4-9).

RED CELL INDICES

The red cell corpuscular values were introduced for the study of anemia. To determine the indices of a red cell count, hemoglobin and hematocrit are necessary (Figure 4-10).

The mean corpuscular volume (MCV) is the average volume, expressed in cubic microns, of the individual red cells.

The mean corpuscular hemoglobin (MCH) is the weight or content of hemoglobin of the average individual red cell in micromicrograms.

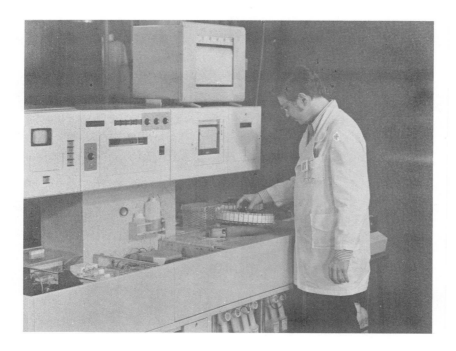

FIGURE 4-9: Hemolog D® machine used in hematology.

In most instances of anemia the average size of the red cells (or MCV) and weight of hemoglobin in the red cells (or MCH) undergo similar changes so that the MCV and MCH would vary from the normal in a similar fashion.

The mean corpuscular hemoglobin concentration (MCHC) expresses as a percentage the average hemoglobin concentration per 100 ml of packed red cells.

The red cell indices are useful in diagnosing the morphologic type of anemia to further pinpoint the diagnosis as microcytic, hypochromic, normochromic, macrocytic, etc.

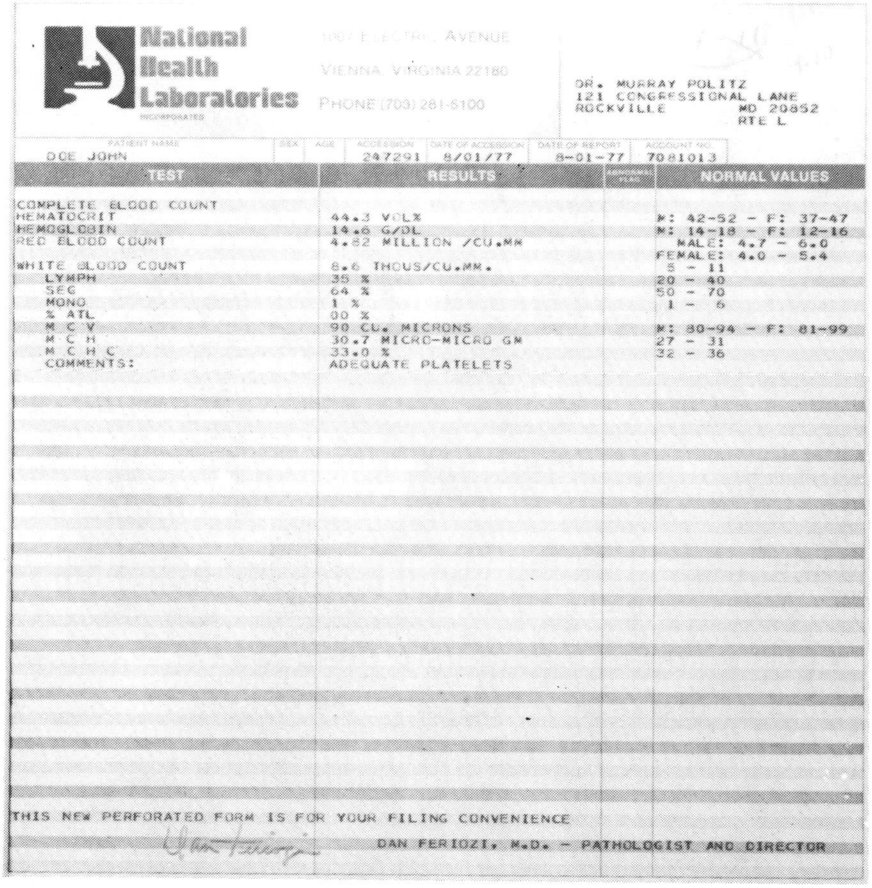

National Health Laboratories
INCORPORATED
[illegible] ELECTRIC AVENUE
VIENNA, VIRGINIA 22180
PHONE (703) 281-6100

DR. MURRAY POLITZ
121 CONGRESSIONAL LANE
ROCKVILLE MD 20852
RTE L

PATIENT NAME	SEX	AGE	ACCESSION	DATE OF ACCESSION	DATE OF REPORT	ACCOUNT NO.
DOE JOHN			247291	8/01/77	8-01-77	7081013

TEST	RESULTS		NORMAL VALUES
COMPLETE BLOOD COUNT			
HEMATOCRIT	44.3 VOL%		M: 42-52 - F: 37-47
HEMOGLOBIN	14.6 G/DL		M: 14-18 - F: 12-16
RED BLOOD COUNT	4.82 MILLION /CU.MM		MALE: 4.7 - 6.0 FEMALE: 4.0 - 5.4
WHITE BLOOD COUNT	8.6 THOUS/CU.MM.		5 - 11
LYMPH	35 %		20 - 40
SEG	64 %		50 - 70
MONO	1 %		1 - 6
% ATL	00 %		
M C V	90 CU. MICRONS		M: 80-94 - F: 81-99
M C H	30.7 MICRO-MICRO GM		27 - 31
M C H C	33.0 %		32 - 36
COMMENTS:	ADEQUATE PLATELETS		

THIS NEW PERFORATED FORM IS FOR YOUR FILING CONVENIENCE

DAN FERIOZI, M.D. - PATHOLOGIST AND DIRECTOR

FIGURE 4-10: Complete blood count with red cell indices. (From National Health Laboratories, Inc., Vienna, Virginia, with permission.)

Typical anemic patterns of morphologic classification* would show the following changes in the indices:

*From Medical Services Company of Arizona: *Quick Reference Laboratory Manual for the Physician*, 1973, p. 70, with permission.

Normocytic	MCV 80-94	MCH 27-32	MCHC 33-38
Macrocytic	MCV 94-160	MCH 32-50	MCHC 32-36
Microcytic	MCV 72-80	MCH 21-24	MCHC 30-70
Microcytic hypochromic	MCV 50-80	MCH 12-29	MCHC 24-30

BLOOD OXYGEN

Molecular oxygen is transported from the lungs to the tissues by blood primarily because of the ability of hemoglobin to combine reversibly with oxygen to form oxyhemoglobin. Four different but related blood oxygen measurements are of clinical significance: they are oxygen content, capacity, saturation, and tension.

The oxygen content is the concentration of oxygen which varies with the hemoglobin concentration of the blood, the presence or absence of pulmonary or circulatory pathology as well as the physiological state with respect to rest or exercise. The oxygen capacity is the maximum quantity of oxygen capable of being held by the blood. Oxygen saturation expresses as a percentage the ratio of the content to the capacity. The quantity of oxygen dissolved and that combined with hemoglobin are dependent on the oxygen tension to which the blood is subjected. When the oxygen tension is high, almost all the hemoglobin combines with oxygen. The amount of oxygen physically dissolved in the plasma is directly proportional to the partial pressure.

ERYTHROCYTE SEDIMENTATION RATE (ESR)

The increased rate at which erythrocytes settle in a given period of time has long been associated with pathologic conditions, especially inflammation. Erythrocytes settle more rapidly in the blood of women than that of men and accelerate further during pregnancy. An increased sedimentation rate has also been noted in chronic infectious diseases such as tuberculosis, in cancer, in collagen disease, in acute localized inflammations along with an increase in leukocytes, and in dysprotein anemias such as multiple myeloma.

Fibrinogen, globulin, and cholesterol accelerate the sedimentation rate whereas an increase in plasma viscosity slows down the rate by counteracting the acceleration effect of blood proteins on rouleaux formation. In anemia, because a change in the erythrocyte plasma ratio favors rouleaux formation, the ESR is accelerated. If the shape of red cells is abnormal or irregular, as in sickle-cell diseases or spherocytosis, and does not allow rouleaux to form, the ESR will be low.

Rouleaux formation is the alignment of red blood cells one upon another resembling a stack of coins. Elevated plasma fibrinogen or globulins cause rouleaux to form and would also increase the sedimentation rate.

WHITE BLOOD CELLS OR LEUKOCYTES

White blood cells are important as part of the body's defense mechanism. The percentage distribution of the different types of leukocytes and the qualitative study of them are performed in a stained smear, usually using Wright's stain (Figure 4-11). Each dif-

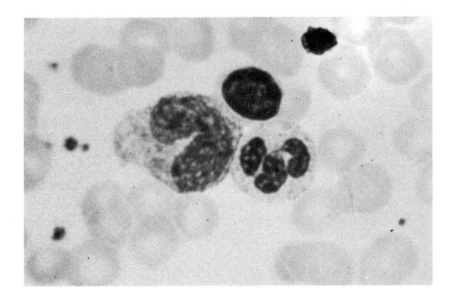

FIGURE 4-11: A neutrophil, lymphocyte and monocyte. (From the Armed Forces Institute of Pathology, Washington, D.C., Negative No. L-12967-46, with permission.)

ferent leukocyte is counted under the microscope, usually using a recording tabulator. One hundred cells are counted by pressing a separate key for each specific cell and the percentage can be read directly as the instrument indicates when a count of one hundred has been reached.

Acute bacterial infections stimulate the production of neutrophils causing a leukocytosis. If destruction exceeds production of white cells, then a normal cell count or even a leukopenia may be seen. Acute viral infections do not stimulate leukopoiesis and may inhibit it, causing a leukopenia (Figure 4-12). On occasion a lymphocytosis may occur.

NEUTROPHILS

Neutrophils have a multiple-lobed nucleus appearing polynuclear. The size averages $12\,\mu$m and the average number of lobes in the nucleus is three, all joined by a thin filament to each other. The

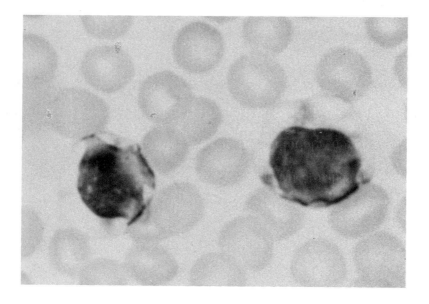

FIGURE 4-12: Atypical lymphocytes in infectious mononucleosis with the "ballerina skirt" effect as seen in viral infections. (From the Armed Forces Institute of Pathology, Washington, D.C., Negative No. L-12967-34, with permission.)

segmented neutrophils constitute 50—70 percent of leukocytes in adults with children having lower normals. Young neutrophils or band neutrophils, defined as lacking a nuclear filament, are normally present in small numbers with up to one third of the neutrophils considered normal. Neutrophils are important in defense against infectious disease. A "shift to the left" occurs when there are increased bands and less mature neutrophils in the blood as well as a lower average in the number of lobes present in segmented cells (Figure 4-13).

LYMPHOCYTES

Lymphocytes are large mononuclear cells without specific cytoplasmic granules. The nucleus is sharply defined and usually round but may be indented on one side. Lymphocytes may be small, 6 to 10 μm, or large, 12 to 20 μm in diameter. The larger ones are frequently found in children, and are difficult to distinguish from monocytes. Lymphocytes constitute from 20 to 40 percent of all leukocytes in

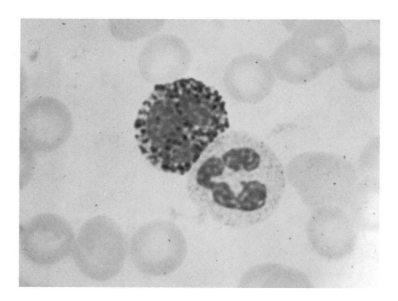

FIGURE 4-13: Segmented neutrophil and basophil. (From the Armed Forces Institute of Pathology, Washington, D.C., Negative No. L-12967-48, with permission.)

adults and 60 percent in the first year of life, decreasing to approximately 36 percent at age 10. Lymphocytes function in cell-mediated immunity, including delayed hypersensitivity, graft rejection, defense against intracellular organisms such as tubercle bacillus, brucella, and neoplasms. They also play a part in the production of antibodies (Figure 4-14).

MONOCYTES

Monocytes are the largest of the blood cells, measuring 14–20 μm in diameter (Figure 4-15). They are mononuclear cells with abundant cytoplasm and the nucleus may be lobulated, deeply indented, or horse-shoe-shaped. Monocytes transform into macrophages, which are larger and ingest and destroy particles or cells including bacteria, Ig6 immunoglobulin or complement, and act as phagocytes in cell-mediated immunity (Figures 4-16 and 4-17).

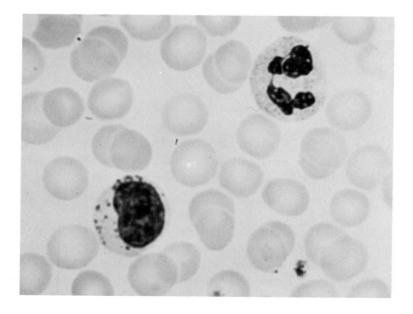

FIGURE 4-14: Lymphocyte and segmented neutrophil. (From the Armed Forces Institute of Pathology, Washington, D.C., Negative No. L-12967-82, with permission.)

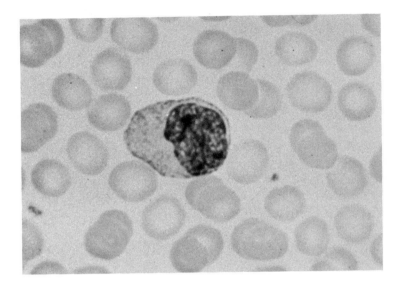

FIGURE 4-15: Monocyte. (From the Armed Forces Institute of Pathology, Washington, D.C., Negative No. L-12967-41, with permission.)

BASOPHILS

Basophils resemble the polymorphonuclear neutrophils except the nucleus is only slightly lobulated or indented and the granules stain a deep purple with Wright's stain. The basophils comprise 0.5 percent or less of the total leukocytes and appear to react in allergic states. They contain about one-half of the blood histamine.

EOSINOPHILS

Eosinophils are similar to the polymorphonuclear neutrophils except for the large granules in the cytoplasm which stain red with eosin-containing stains. The nucleus rarely contains more than three segments whereas neutrophils may contain five. The eosinophils comprise from one to five percent of the leukocytes. They respond late in inflammation and are attracted to antigen-antibody complexes which they phagocytize. They carry about one-third of the blood histamine (Figure 4-18).

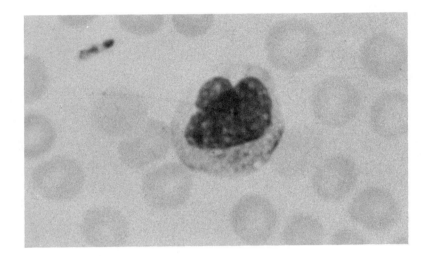

FIGURE 4-16: Monocyte in infectious mononucleosis. (From the Armed Forces Institute of Pathology, Washington, D.C., Negative No. L-12967-24, with permission.)

MYELOCYTES

Myelocytes are immature neutrophic granulocytes which have not developed into mature or early cells. They are not normally seen in circulation and may be found along with metamyelocytes in conditions such as pernicious anemia, myelocytic leukemia, and a leukocytosis which may be exceedingly high due to multiple etiologies (Figure 4-19).

WHITE BLOOD CELL COUNT

In the total white blood cell count no effort is made to differentiate the normal cell types which comprise the leukocytes. The normal range for the count in an adult is 4,500—11,000/μl.

Manual leukocyte counting is rarely performed because of the excellent and efficient electronic counting chambers. The same prin-

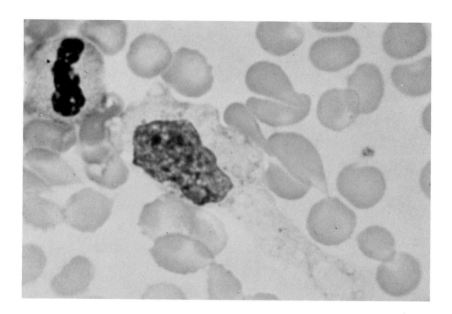

FIGURE 4-17: A large monocyte cell (macrophage) with a long pseudopod is suggestive of subacute bacterial endocarditis. (From the Armed Forces Institute of Pathology, Washington, D.C., Negative No. L-12967-57, with permission.)

ciples for counting apply to the white cells as were described for the red cells except the red cells in this instance are lysed before counting occurs.

The white cell count of children through adolescence is higher than that of an adult. It ranges from 15,500 cells per cu/mm in infants and 13,000 cells per cu/mm in adolescents. Children usually run a lymphocytosis of 40—50 percent.

Neutrophilia

Neutrophilia is an increase in the neutrophils which may be caused by:

1. Infection:

Neutrophilia may be seen in typhoid fever, paratyroid fever, and brucellosis. Usually in infection there is a charac-

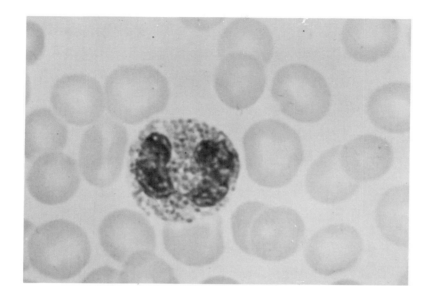

FIGURE 4-18: Eosinophil. (From the Armed Forces Institute of Pathology, Washington, D.C., Negative No. L-12967-49, with permission.)

teristic shift to the left with a fall in eosinophils and a neutrophilic leukocytosis with an increase in young forms. When the infection subsides and the fever drops the total number of leukocytes decreases, the monocytes increase and are gradually replaced with a lymphocytosis and eosinophilia.

2. Toxic conditions or agents:
   (a) metabolic uremia, eclampsia, gout, diabetic acidosis.
   (b) drugs and chemicals—lead, mercury, potassium, chloride, digitalis, epinephrine, corticosteroids, turpentine, ethylene glycol, benzene.
3. physical and emotional stimuli—heat, cold, pain, fear, etc.
4. tissue destruction or necrosis, burns, surgery, injury, fractures.
5. hemorrhage.
6. hemolysis.
7. hematologic disorders—leukemia, post-splenectomy.

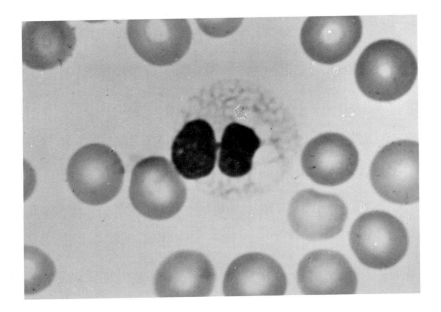

FIGURE 4-19: Atypical segmented neutrophil in myelocytic leukemia. (From the Armed Forces Institute of Pathology, Washington, D.C., Negative No. L-12967-3, with permission.)

Neutropenia

Neutropenia is a decrease in neutrophils which may be caused by:

1. myeloid hypoplasia.
2. ineffective granulocytopoiesis.
3. decreased survival rate in circulation.
4. lupus erythematosus, shock, typhoid, malaria, paratyphoid fever.
5. drugs.
6. vitamin B_{12} and folic acid deficiency.

Eosinophilia

Eosinophilia is an increase in eosinophils which may be caused by:

1. allergic states.
2. skin disorders such as eczema.
3. parasitic infestations.
4. infectious diseases.
5. blood diseases such as leukemia.
5. splenectomy.

Eosinopenia

Eosinopenia is a decrease in eosinophils which may be caused by:

1. severe infections with neutrophilia.
2. Cushing's syndrome.
3. electric shock therapy.
4. after injection of ACTH or epinephrine.

Basophilia

Basophilia is an increase in basophils which may be caused by:

1. allergic reactions.
2. chronic granulocytic leukemia.
3. myeloid metaplasia.
4. polycythemia vera.

Basopenia

Basopenia is a decrease in basophils which may be caused by:

1. acute infections.
2. ACTH or corticosteroids.

Because of their rarity a disease is not readily detected.

Lymphyocytosis

Lymphocytosis is an increase in lymphocytes which may be

caused by many conditions where there is a neutropenia such as:

1. German measles.
2. brucellosis.
3. congenital syphilis.
4. thyrotoxicosis.
5. pertussis.
6. mononucleosis.

Lymphocytopenia

Lymphocytopenia is a decrease in lymphocytes caused by:

1. Hodgkin's disease.
2. drugs or irradiation.
3. adrenocortical hormones.
4. immunological deficiency disorders.

Monocytosis

Monocytosis is an increase in monocytes which may be caused by:

1. recovery from acute infections.
2. subacute bacterial endocarditis.
3. mycotic, rickettsial, protozoal and viral infections.
4. hematologic disease.
5. leukemia.
6. Hodgkin's disease.

Plasmacytosis

This is an increase in plasma cells which are not normally present in circulatory blood. The plasma cells are increased in chronic infection, allergic states, neoplastic conditions, and in conditions in which the serum gamma globulin is elevated. They may be moderately elevated in infectious mononucleosis, syphilis, subacute bacterial endocarditis, sarcoidosis and collagen diseases. Their increase is usually associated with an increase of lymphocytes, monocytes, and eosinophils. These four cells form the antigen-antibody quartet. In marrow they are decreased or absent in agammaglobulinemia.

LEUKEMIA

Leukemia is a generalized neoplastic proliferation of leuko-poietic cells with or without peripheral blood involvement. Leukemia may be acute, subacute, or chronic. As cell types they may be classed as undifferentiated blast cell leukemia, granulocytic leukemia, lymphocytic leukemia, monocytic leukemia, plasma cell leukemia and lymphosarcoma leukemia. An absence of elevated total leuko-cytes with the presence of abnormal cells is called subleukemic leukemia. Aleukemic leukemia is the term used when no abnormal cells are present (Figures 4-20 and 4-21).

LEUKEMOID REACTION

Leukemoid reaction is an excessive leukocytosis to a stimulus that normally would result in a smaller increase in the number of leukocytes or immaturity in the cells. A 50,000 per µl count or higher

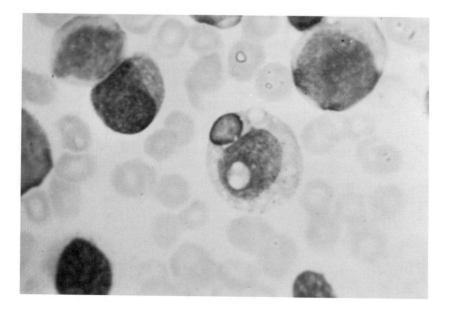

FIGURE 4-20: Monocyte in acute monocytic leukemia. (From the Armed Forces Institute of Pathology, Washington, D.C., Negative No. L-12967-4, with permission.)

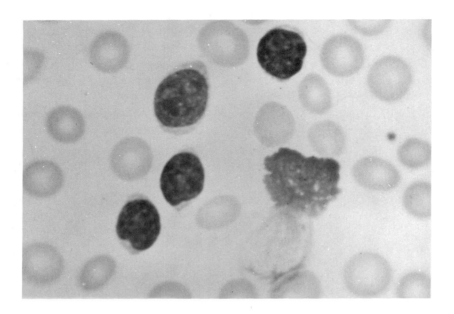

FIGURE 4-21: Lymphocytes in lymphocytic leukemia. (From the Armed Forces Institute of Pathology, Washington, D.C., Negative No. L-12967-50, with permission.)

with a shift to the left or a lower count (even lower than normal) with considerable immature leukocytes, is present. Leukemoid reaction may be neutrophilic, eosinophilic, lymphocytic, or monocytic in nature and may be seen in hemolytic crisis, hemorrhage, Hodgkin's disease, various infections, burns, eclampsia, mustard-gas poisoning, vascular thrombosis or infarction, neoplasm in bone marrow and myeloid metaplasia (Figure 4-22).

PLATELETS

Platelets are round or oval usually 2—4 μm in diameter, but may be larger if production is increased or post-splenectomy. Platelet counts may vary considerably in number in many instances. Newborns during the first two days have fewer platelets than older infants. The number of platelets decrease before menstruation and begin to rise the day of onset. Platelet counts are high after violent ex-

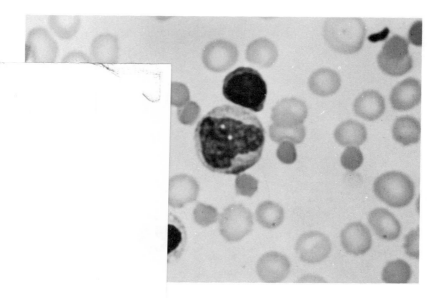

monocyte and neutrophilic leukocyte are noted. The
 a diagnosis of hemolytic anemia secondary to
clostridium perfringens septicemia. (From the Armed Forces Institute of Pathology,
Washington, D.C., Negative No. L-12967-105, with permission.)

ercise, higher altitude ascension, and in winter rather than summer
months. The mature megakaryocyte produces platelets as shed cytoplasmic fragments (Figure 4-23). One third of the platelets are always
in the spleen so that in splenomegaly up to 80—90 percent may be
within the spleen resulting in a thrombocytopenia. Platelets function
in supporting the endothelium of blood vessels. In severe thrombocytopenia, tiny hemorrhages known as petechiae occur from vascular
leaks (Figure 4-24). In hemostasis, platelets adhere to collagen in a
damaged vessel and clump together to form a plug in an attempt to
stop blood from leaving the injured vessel.

Platelet Count

Platelets are the smallest of formed elements in the blood with a

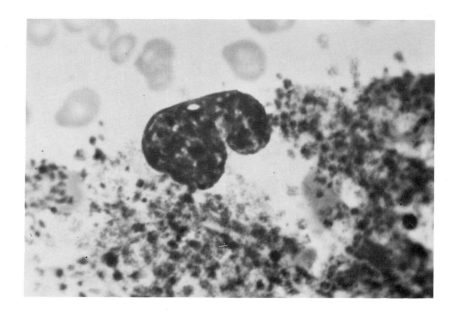

FIGURE 4-23: Aggregates of thrombocytes surrounding the nucleus of a megakaryocyte. (From the Armed Forces Institute of Pathology, Washington, D.C., Negative No. L-12967-80, with permission.)

range of 150,000−400,000 µl. They function in hemostasis and also in maintaining vascular integrity. They are difficult to distinguish from debris because of their size and also tend to adhere to glass and each other. An estimate of their numbers and size should be included in a laboratory report from a slide made of venous blood with EDTA.

Thrombocythemia

Thrombocythemia is a condition in which the platelet count is persistently elevated to levels at least three times normal. This disorder may be part of a general proliferative disorder such as polycythemia vera and chronic granulocytic leukemia, or it may be part of a hematologic disorder such as a bleeding problem. Thrombocythemia is easily recognized by an increase in platelets of .9−14 million per µl with abnormal and giant forms usually present. Neutro-

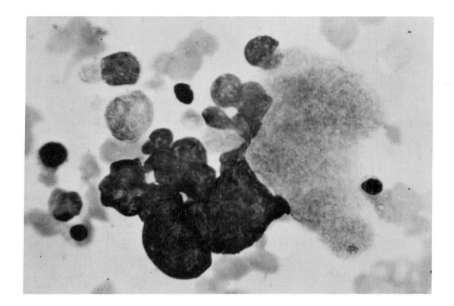

FIGURE 4-24: A large, mechanically traumatized megakaryocyte with no evidence of thrombocyte production from the bone marrow of a patient with thrombotic thrombocytopenic purpura. (From the Armed Forces Institute of Pathology, Washington, D.C., Negative No. L-12967-83, with permission.)

philic leukocytosis is usually present, and microcytic anemia due to chronic blood loss may be found.

Thrombocytosis

Thrombocytosis is an increase in platelets above 400,000 per μl. Platelet production increases in situations such as iron deficiency, acute hemorrhage, hemolysis, inflammatory diseases, and malignancies. Loss of splenic function or splenectomy removes the site where one-third of platelets reside and results in thrombocytosis.

Administration of epinephrine will also result in thrombocytosis as will myeloproliferative diseases in extramedullary sites and marrow caused by altered distribution, increased destruction or decreased production. If severe, abnormal bleeding may occur. The bleeding time is a test of both platelet number and function.

ANEMIA

Anemia is a state in which red blood cell values are less than normal. It is defined as a condition in which the blood is deficient either in quantity (oligogemia) or in quality. The deficiency in quality may consist of a diminution in the amount of hemoglobin (oligochromemia) or in diminution in the number of red blood corpuscles (oligocythemia) or both.

Anemia signifies a reduction in the amount of oxygen-carrying hemoglobin in a given volume of blood. The normal corpuscle circulates in the blood stream for about 120 days before it fragments in the circulation or is phagocyted primarily in the spleen. The balance between formation and destruction is finely balanced and totals about 9 billion per hour or 0.8 percent of the red blood cells per day.

BASIC LABORATORY TESTS FOR DIAGNOSIS

When anemia is discovered the basic laboratory procedures should include:
  a. Hemoglobin
  b. Hematocrit
  c. RBC with indices
  d. Blood film examination
  e. WBC
  f. Platelet count
  g. Reticulocyte count.

The anemias may be classified as either etiologic or morphologic.

ETIOLOGIC CLASSIFICATION

1. Blood loss.
2. Excessive destruction of red corpuscles.
3. Impaired production of red corpuscles principally caused by:
  a. Deficiency of substances essential for erythropoiesis (iron, vitamin B_{12}, folic acid, protein deficiency)
  b. Endocrine deficiency (pituitary, thyroid, adrenal, or testicular hormones)
  c. Physical or chemical injury (radiation, benzol, lead, and various other bone marrow toxins)
  d. Myelophthisic anemias (leukemia, Hodgkin's disease, mye-

lofibrosis, malignancy with metastases, granulomatous involvement of marrow)
    e. Anemia associated with splenic disorders
    f. Idiopathic bone marrow failure.

MORPHOLOGIC CLASSIFICATION

1. Macrocytic
    a. Megaloblastic (deficiency of vitamin B_{12} or folic acid)
    b. Miscellaneous such as chronic liver disease, hypothyroidism, normocytic anemias made temporarily macrocytic.
2. Normocytic
    a. Sudden loss of blood
    b. Hemolytic anemias
    c. Anemias caused principally by impaired production (except deficiencies of vitamin B_{12}, folic acid and iron)
3. Microcytic normochromic
    a. A subacute and chronic inflammatory condition affecting the red cell formation.
4. Microcytic hypochromic
    a. Iron deficiency anemia
    b. Miscellaneous.

Hypochromic Anemia

Hypochromic anemia almost always means iron deficiency. Dietary deficiency is rare in adults; however, it may occur in malabsorption syndrome, thalassemia, and achlorhydria. Pregnancy may also exhibit this type of anemia due to an increased demand for iron. With inadequate iron supplies, a drop occurs in hemoglobin and hematocrit. The red cells have a decreased amount of hemoglobin and are small (microcytic) and pale (hypochromic). The mean corpuscular hemoglobin concentration is less than 30 percent and the mean corpuscular volume is less than 80 microns.

Idiopathic Steatorrhea

Idiopathic steatorrhea, in which the intestinal wall is unable to absorb folic acid, vitamin B_{12}, or iron, causes a depletion of the body stores of these substances. Folic acid is necessary for the maturation of granulocytes and megakaryocytes, and deficiency may cause a leukopenia and thrombocytopenia as well as hyperchromic and macrocytic red cells. The neutrophils are hypersegmented as in pernicious anemia. This clinical picture may also be seen in malnutrition, in pregnancy, and in drug reactions such as anticonvulsants like diphenylhydantoin. If iron is poorly absorbed, a microcytic, hypochromic anemia will be seen.

Pernicious Anemia

Pernicious anemia, in which vitamin B_{12} is not absorbed because the cells of the gastric mucosa are unable to produce the intrinsic factor of Castle, causes a liver depletion of B_{12} and a disturbance in the production of DNA. The hemoglobin and hematocrit decrease because fewer red blood cells are released into the circulation from the bone marrow. The cells that are released are macrocytic and hyperchromic. They are of various sizes (anisocytosis) and shapes (poikilocytosis) (Figure 4-25). The serum bilirubin may be elevated

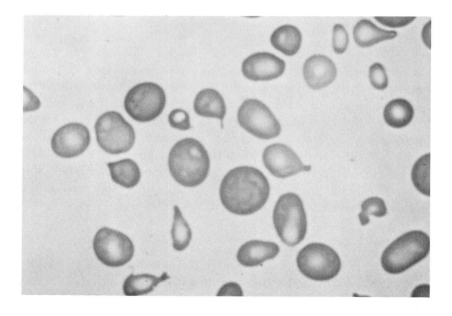

FIGURE 4-25: Anisocytosis and poikilocytosis of erythrocytes in pernicious anemia. (From the Armed Forces Institute of Pathology, Washington, D.C., Negative No. L-12967-112, with permission.)

since their life span is short. Because of the DNA synthesis disturbance the maturation of granulocytes and megakaryocytes is affected, leading to a leukopenia and thrombocytopenia. The serum
iron may be elevated because of the decreased utilization of iron for
red cell synthesis. Definitive diagnosis should include a gastric
analysis and Schilling Test (Figure 4-26).

Sickle-Cell Anemia

Sickle-cell anemia is seen in one in six-hundred American
Negroes and is named after the sickle-shaped cells seen in venous
blood. The presence of Hgb-S or sickle-cell hemoglobin is responsible for most of the symptoms of the disease. The anemia present is
normochromic and red-cell counts may be in the range of 2.5 million
per cu/mm. Target cells, polychromasia, occasional sickled erythrocytes, numerous nucleated red cells and a mild leukocytosis are present in the morphologic studies (Figure 4-27).

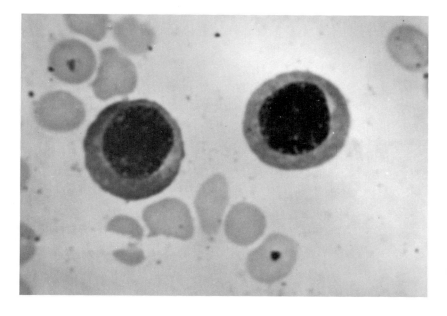

FIGURE 4-26: Two nucleated red cells which are abnormally large (macrocytic or
megaloblastic) in pernicious anemia. (From the Armed Forces Institute of
Pathology, washington, D.C., Negative No. L-12967-11, with permission.)

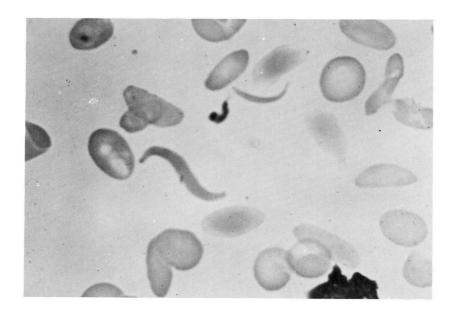

FIGURE 4-27: Sickle cells in sickle-cell anemia. (From the Armed Forces Institute of Pathology, Washington, D.C.,Negative No. L-12967-113, with permission.)

POLYCYTHEMIA VERA

Polycythemia vera presents a picture of an increase in red blood cells with an increase in hematocrit and hemoglobin. The cells are normal in appearance. The platelets are usually increased and a leukocytosis is also present with a shift to the left. The uric acid level is also commonly elevated.

CHAPTER 5

Hemostasis

DEFINITION AND PHASES OF HEMOSTASIS

Hemostasis is the process whereby the escape of blood from the vascular tree is stopped or prevented. There are many phases of normal hemostasis and they may overlap. The phases include:

A. Vascular Phase
B. Platelet Phase
C. Blood Coagulation
D. Clot Retraction
E. Fibrinolysis
F. Repair

There are numerous body safeguards to prevent abnormal bleeding. The vascular integrity is probably of prime importance. After injury, the local flow of blood decreases due to the reflex vasoconstriction of arterioles and metarterioles. Platelets (discussed in Chapter 4) aggregate at the site of injury and release vasoconstrictor catecholamines and serotonin which help with vasoconstriction. Also released are glucocorticoids, procoagulators, and a protein that retracts the fibrin mass. Inhibition of excessive coagulation by anticoagulants and dissolution of the clot in the repair phase completes the cycle.

Blood coagulation has received more attention than any other phase of hemostasis and still remains fairly confusing. The classic theory for the process of blood coagulation is:

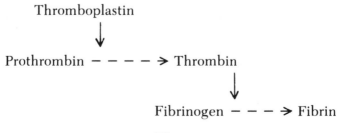

57

MECHANISM

The mechanism of blood clotting may be divided into three stages.

Stage 1.   The production of plasma (extrinsic) or tissue (intrinsic) thromboplastin to form prothrombin activator.

Stage 2.   The conversion of prothrombin to thrombin by thromboplastin.

Stage 3.   The conversion of fibrinogen to fibrin by the proteolytic action of thrombin. Calcium is required in all stages.

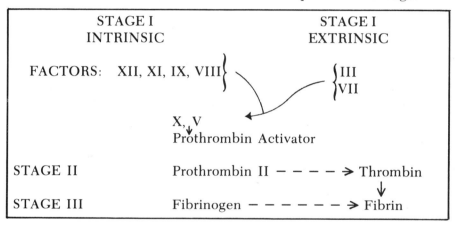

NOMENCLATURE

The international nomenclature for blood coagulation factors is as follows:

Factor I.   Fibrinogen
Factor II.   Prothrombin
Factor III.   Tissue Thromboplastin
Factor IV.   Calcium
Factor V.   Labile Factor
Factor VII.   Stable Factor
Factor VIII.   Antihemophilic Globulin
Factor IX.   Plasma thromboplastin component (Christmas Factor)
Factor X.   Stuart—Prower Factor
Factor XI.   Plasma Thromoplastin Antecedent
Factor XII.   Hageman Factor

CLINICAL SIGNS

In clinical laboratory diagnosis, attention should be given to the character of the bleeding. Petechiae indicate platelet or blood vessel defects. Ecchymosis and hematomas are usually caused by coagulation defects in addition to platelet and blood vessel abnormalities. Hemarthroses are most commonly seen in severe coagulation abnormalities such as hemophilia. Purpuric lesions are usually asymptomatic; however, if they are accompanied by paresthesias, pain, a vasculitis or autoerythrocyte sensitization may be the cause.

TESTS

Plasma is a reagent in most tests used to evaluate clotting. This is obtained by adding calcium binding anticoagulant solutions with whole blood. Plasma obtained by this means can be studied by the addition of sufficient calcium to neutralize the anticoagulant which was added. Solutions utilized for this purpose are sodium oxylate, sodium citrate, EDTA and occasionally heparin.

BLEEDING TIME

Bleeding time is the duration of bleeding from a standard puncture-wound of the skin and tests the function of platelets as well as the integrity of the vessel wall.

    A. *Duke Method:* The ear lobe is punctured and the time is noted after blotting with friction paper every 30 seconds until blood no longer stains the paper. Normal is 6—10 minutes.

    B. *Ivy Method:* A blood-pressure cuff is put on the arm above the elbow and inflated to 40 mm Hg. The forearm is punctured and blotted every 30 seconds until no stain is on the paper. Normal is 2—3 minutes.

CLOTTING TIME

Clotting time is the time taken for whole blood to form a solid clot when removed from the vascular system and exposed to a foreign substance.

    A. *Lee White:* Blood is collected in test tubes which are then immersed in a water bath (37°C) and are tilted every 15 seconds. When no blood flows down the side of the tube because of a solid clot, the tube is marked. Normal is 5—8 minutes.

3. *Capillary Method:* Two plain capillary-tubes are filled with blood (usually obtained from earlobe puncture) and the stopwatch is started as soon as the puncture is made. Every 30 seconds, a portion of one of the filled capillary-tubes is broken and checked for the presence of a fibrin clot. The time required for the presence of the fibrin strand is the clotting time. By the capillary method, the normal time is 2—6 minutes.

PARTIAL THROMBOPLASTIN TIME

Certain thromboplastins, lacking the ability to compensate for the plasma defect of hemophilia, are called partial thromboplastins. The test will be abnormal with a significant plasma deficiency of any procoagulants other than Factors VII and XIII. The same sample can be used for a Prothrombin Time or a P.T. The P.T.T. (or Partial Thromboplastin Time) should be within 5 seconds of the control time. Any result over 20 seconds longer than the control is abnormal and shows a deficiency of one of the plasma procoagulants or is the result of heparin therapy.

PROTHROMBIN TIME

Plasma from blood in which a calcium-binding anticoagulant has been added will coagulate when calcium is added in the presence of tissue thromboplastin. The time between the addition of calcium and the presence of a visible clot is the Prothrombin Time. Normal plasma will clot in about 12 seconds following the addition of calcium with a potent tissue thromboplastin. The Prothrombin Time will be long with deficiencies of prothrombin, Factor V, Factor II or Factor X. Often the protime may be expressed as a percent of activity relative to a control sample based on time elapsed for a clot to form. This stage is affected by Coumadin®° type anticoagulants.

TOURNIQUET TEST

Capillary fragility is measured by mounting pressure halfway between systolic and diastolic for a standard time interval. The lack

°Endo Laboratories, Garden City, New York

of appearance of petechiae is an indication of normal vascular integrity.

The appearance of minute subcutaneous hemorrhages below the area at which a rubber bandage is applied not too tightly for ten minutes upon the upper arm, characteristic of scarlet fever and hemorrhagic diathesis, is known as the Rumpel-Leede phenomenon.

CHAPTER 6

Urine Analysis

SPECIMEN COLLECTION

Preoperative laboratory tests performed on patients should include a urinalysis. This chapter will review many of the usual results of urinalysis and includes more specific diagnostic tests. For the usual preoperative test, a random voided specimen of urine is satisfactory. The examination should be performed thirty minutes after collection; if this is not possible, refrigeration of the specimen is mandatory. In routine urinalysis the laboratories usually perform tests and report results for color, appearance, reaction, specific gravity, glucose, albumin, acetone, W.B.C., R.B.C., epithelial cells, bacteria, crystals and casts (Figure 6-1).

COLOR

Normal color for urine varies from straw to amber usually being reported as yellow. Colorless will mean a reduction in the concentration of urine. Yellow foam may indicate bile or certain medication reactions. A milky appearance may mean the presence of bacteria, epithelial cells or frank pus. A smoky-brown to reddish color indicates blood. Port wine color may indicate the presence of porphorins. A black discoloration may be indicative of melanin. Orange, blue, or red may indicate medications.

APPEARANCE

The appearance of urine may be classed as cloudy or clear. Some normal causes of cloudiness may be crystals or epithelial cells. In disease conditions, the principal causes of cloudiness may be pus, blood, bacteria, and casts. Urine has a faintly aromatic odor. Odor is chiefly important in the recognition of specimens that, due to bacterial contamination on standing, become fetid. Characteristic odors are present after ingestion of asparagus or thyme, and in maple-syrup urine disease, phenylketoneuria, and certain metabolic disorders.

	ACCOUNT NO.	SPECIMEN NO.
	00000000	12-17-0007

DATE OF SPECIMEN	DATE PROCESSED	SEX	AGE
12 OCT 76	13 OCT 76	M	44

REPORT
Biomedical
Laboratories, Inc.

LAST   FIRST   PATIENT NAME   MIDDLE
DOE JOHN

PATIENT ADDRESS
1610 MAPLE AVE
ALEXANDRIA VA 22311

PHYSICIAN OR LABORATORY
DR MURRAY J POLITZ
ROCKVILLE MD 20852

ADDITIONAL INFORMATION

LABORATORY REGISTER NO. 289

TEST	RESULT	LIMITS
20271		
COLOR	YELLOW.	YELLOW
APPEARANCE	CLEAR	CLEAR
SPECIFIC GRAVITY	1.014	1.010-1.030
PH	6	5-7
GLUCOSE	NEGATIVE	NEGATIVE
PROTEIN	NEGATIVE	NEGATIVE
OCCULT BLOOD	NEGATIVE	NEGATIVE
ACETONE	NEGATIVE	NEGATIVE
WBC/HPF	NONE	
RBC/HPF	NONE	
EPITHELIAL CELLS	MODERATE	
CASTS	NONE	
CRYSTALS	NONE	
SEDIMENTATION RATE	5 MM/HR	5-20
VDRL, SERUM	NON-REACTIVE	NON-REACTIVE
COMPLETED REPORT		

| CALCIUM | PHOSPHORUS | GLUCOSE | UREA | URIC ACID | CHOLESTEROL | PROTEIN | ALBUMIN | BILIRUBIN | ALKALINE | LDH | SGOT |
					TOTAL	TOTAL		TOTAL	PHOSPHATASE		
		72	15	4.8	299H						
mg/DL	mg/DL	mg/DL	mg/DL	(M 2.5-8.0)	mg/DL	g/DL	g/DL	mg/DL	mIU/ml	mIU/ml	mIU/ml
(8.5-10.5)	(2.5-4.5)	(50-110)	(10-20)	(F 2.5-6.4)	(150-300)	(6.0-8.0)	(3.5-5.5)	(0.1-1.0)	(20-115)	(100-225)	(5-40)

| T4 BY | T3 UPTAKE | THYROXINE | BILIRUBIN | THYMOL | WBC | RBC | HGB | HCT | MCV | MCH | MCHC |
RIA		FREE	DIRECT	TURBIDITY	x 10³/mm³	x 10⁶/mm³	g/DL	%	µ³	µµg	%
					5.8	4.65	15.6	45.7	98	33.3H	34.1
mg/DL	(M 40-62)	mg/DL	mg/DL	units	M 4.8-10.8	M 4.7-6.1	M 14.0-18.0	M 42-52	M 80-94	M 27-31	M 32-36
(4-12)	(F 38-58)	(0.5-2.5)	(0.2-0.25)	(0-6)	F 4.8-10.8	F 4.2-5.4	F 12.0-16.0	F 37-47	F 81-99	F 27-31	F 32-36

| POLYS | BANDS | LYMPHS | MONOS | EOS | BASOS | PLATELET | BLOOD | Rh TYPE | ART | ANTIBODY | RUBELLA TITER |
55-75%	2-5%	25-40%	1-9%	1-4%	1%	ESTIMATION	GROUP		(FOR SYPHILIS)	SCREEN	< 1:6=NO
51		44	4		1	ADEQ					IMMUNITY

FIGURE 6-1: Urinalysis. (From Biomedical Laboratories, Inc., Alexandria, Virginia, with permission.)

REACTION

Reaction of urine refers to the pH range. The pH of urine is the reflection of the ability of the kidney to maintain normal hydrogen-ion concentration in plasma and extracellular fluid. The normal pH is 6 and may vary from 4.6 to 8. Acid urine may be produced by a diet high in meat protein, some fruits, and in pathological states such as renal tubular acidosis and metabolic acidosis. Other causes of acid urine may be found in fever and diabetes, gout, chronic nephritis, acute articular rheumatism, leukemia, and saccharin ingestion.

Alkaline urine may be produced by a diet of certain fruits and vegetables, especially citrus fruits. Alkalinity may also be seen in alkali therapy, retention of urine, blood transfusions, vomiting, and prolonged cold baths. Certain antibiotics work on urinary tract infections better in an alkaline medium which may be induced by sodium bicarbonate or potassium citrate. If allowed to stand, acid urine becomes alkaline because of the decomposition of urea which liberates ammonia.

SPECIFIC GRAVITY

Specific gravity of urine is the term used to compare the weight of urine with the weight of water. Urine, because of its dissolved substances, weighs more than water. In the test, water is given the specific gravity of 1.000. The specific gravity of urine will range between 1.008−1.030. The measurement of the specific gravity of urine is one of the convenient methods of measuring the degree of reabsorptive powers of the kidney. Diseases causing increased water loss from the kidney will dilute the urine specimen, and will therefore lower the specific gravity. A lower specific gravity will be found in individuals with a large fluid intake, chronic nephritis, diabetes insipidus, and primary aldosteronism. An increase in specific gravity may occur in diabetes mellitus, dehydration, sweating, acute glomerulonephritis and fever (Figure 6-2).

GLUCOSE

Glucose and other carbohydrates are normally found in the urine; they are, however, found in quantities that are often too small to be measured by the usual tests. Significant elevations need to be evaluated closely. The presence of larger quantities of urinary glucose, called glycosuria, may occur as a temporary condition following general anesthesia, in pregnancy, and after the administration of certain drugs; however, diabetes is the chief pathologic cause of elevated urinary glucose and it is often best to correlate this with serum glucose levels to gain the most information, especially in diabetes mellitus. Other reasons for increased glycosuria are hyperthyroidism, hyperpituitarism and renal glycosuria.

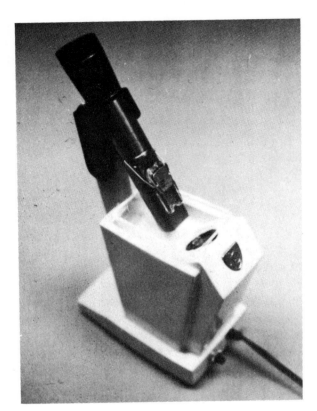

FIGURE 6-2: Urinalysis refractometer for testing specific gravity of urine.

ALBUMIN

Albumin, which is a protein, when found in urine is known as albuminuria. Another term would be proteinuria. Small amounts of protein may be found in urine, but are usually undetected. A "false positive" albuminuria may be caused by excessive exercise, blood from the bladder, vaginal discharge and infections of the urinary track. A sufficient number of pus cells, prostatic secretion, and red blood cells in large enough quantities may also cause a false albuminuria. A true positive albuminuria points to a deficiency in the filtering system of the kidneys and is an aid in the diagnosis of renal disorders. Albuminuria may be found in nephritis, nephrosis, nephrosclerosis, and may also be found in other disease processes with kidney involvement such as amyloidosis, diabetes mellitus, and lupus erythematosus. Bence-Jones Protein found in urine usually indicates the presence of multiple myeloma and may occasionally be seen in leukemia and other malignant bone conditions.

ACETONE

Acetone is not normally found in urine. The acid or ketone bodies are comprised of aceto-acetate, beta hydroxy-butyrate and acetone which are intermediates in the metabolic oxidation of fat. They accumulate in the blood and are excreted in the urine when glucose metabolism is impaired, resulting in acidosis. Typical situations in which ketone bodies are found would include diabetes mellitus and starvation. Acetone is also found in the urine when there is eclampsia, cachexia, fever, and vomiting, and some digestive disorders.

MICROSCOPIC EXAMINATION

The following tests are also included under routine urinalysis; however, they are performed by microscopic examination of the urinary sediments. These sediments are examined under either high- or low-power magnification with an explanation next to the results.

WHITE BLOOD CELLS (W.B.C.)

White blood cells, which may indicate pus in the urine, may also be known as W.B.C. A few W.B.C.'s may be found in normal urine; however, in larger quantities white blood cells may indicate pus in the urine and may be caused by inflammation in the urethra, bladder, kidneys, or in the vagina.

RED BLOOD CELLS (R.B.C.)

Red blood cells should not be found in normal urine and would indicate bleeding from the bladder, ureters, or kidneys. During menses, it should also be noted that contamination from the vagina will cause the presence of R.B.C.'s and should be noted by the podiatrist at the time the test is taken.

EPITHELIAL CELLS

Epithelial cells may normally be seen in the urine and should not be a major concern unless there are many of them together with bacteria and casts which would be indicative of renal disease.

BACTERIA

Bacteria in the urine may be an indication of infection. A few bacteria may be seen in normal urine; however, they are usually seen in bacterial infections of the urethra, bladder, or vagina. Bacteria are reported in the test as +1 +2 +3 +4 depending on the numbers present.

CRYSTALS

Crystals reported in urine seem to be one area of confusion to podiatrists. For this reason, a rather lengthy explanation of the different crystals found in urine is given below.

Ammonium magnesium phosphate crystals found in urine may be prism- or star-shaped and are abundant in pathologic conditions including retention of urine in the bladder, paraplegia, chronic cystitis, enlarged prostate, and chronic pyelitis.

Calcium oxalate crystals are octahedral and dumbbell-shaped. They are found in acid normal urines but are increased in diabetes mellitus, organic liver disease, and heart and lung diseases.

Calcium phosphate crystals are wedge-shaped, often in rosette arrangements, and are found abundantly in pathologic conditions including rention of urine in the bladder, paraplegia, chronic cystitis, enlarged prostate and chronic pyelitis.

Calcium sulfate crystals are large thin needles or prisms found only in acid urine and are of no clinical importance.

Calcium carbonate crystals are dumbbell-shaped crystals like calcium oxalate found mainly in alkaline urine; of no clinical significance.

Uric acid crystals have different shapes and forms, and generally are found in acid urine with a brownish-red color. Their presence does not indicate any pathologic condition. The pathologic conditions they are found in include gout, acute febrile conditions, and chronic nephritis.

Cystine crystals are rarely found in urinary sediments and may produce concretion in the bladder.

Cholesterol crystals appear as colorless plates and may be found in pathologic conditions which include cystitis, pyelitis, chyluria, and nephritis.

Hippuric acid crystals appear as needles or prisms and are pigmented like uric acid crystals. They have no clinical significance.

Leucine and tyromine crystals are highly refractive spherical masses and have been found in pathologic conditions including acute yellow atrophy of the liver, acute phosphorus poisoning, cirrhosis of the liver, severe cases of typhoid fever, and smallpox and leukemia.

Urates may appear as ammonium, calcium, magnesium, potassium and sodium urates in acid urines. Ammonium urate crystals may appear in neutral, alkaline, or acid urines and may appear in pathologic conditions such as gout, acute febrile conditions, and chronic nephritis (Figures 6-3 to 6-6).

CASTS

Casts are molds of the tubule and occur because of "gelling" of the protein. Casts are precipitated in urines of low pH and specific gravity. They may be absent in chronic renal disease even though proteinuria is significant because the capacity to form acid and concentrate urine has been lost.

Hyaline casts are precipitated protein without formed elements.

Epithelial casts are composed largely of desquamated epithelial cells as a result of intrinsic renal disease.

In W.B.C. casts, the cells become emulsed in the protein matrix

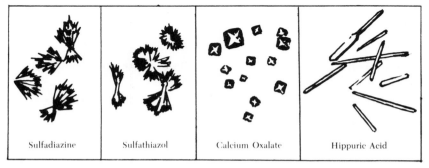

| Sulfadiazine | Sulfathiazol | Calcium Oxalate | Hippuric Acid |

FIGURE 6-3: Crystals in acid, neutral, or slightly alkaline urine.

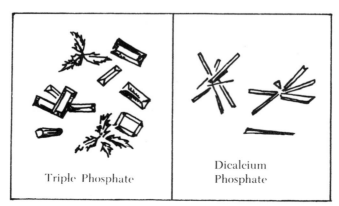

FIGURE 6-4: Crystals in alkaline,neutral, or slightly acid urine.

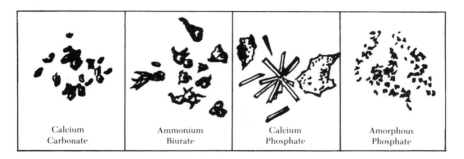

FIGURE 6-5: Crystals in alkaline urine.

and may be found in pyelonephritis or acute glomerulonephritis or systemic lupus erythemotosus.

The cells in red blood cell casts are emulsed in protein matrix and are red-orange in color. These casts are indicative of glomerulitis.

Granular casts are the result of degenerated epithelial cells,

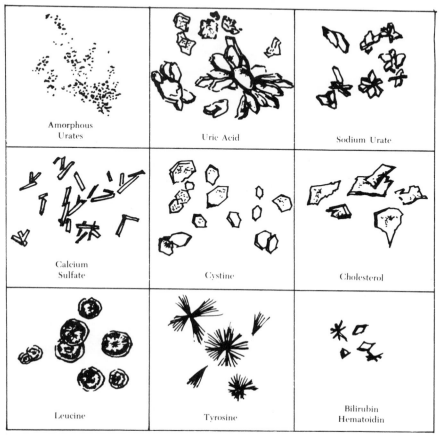

Amorphous Urates	Uric Acid	Sodium Urate
Calcium Sulfate	Cystine	Cholesterol
Leucine	Tyrosine	Bilirubin Hematoidin

FIGURE 6-6: Crystals in acid urine.

W.B.C. or R.B.C. casts and protein which have been in the tubule and not excreted immediately. They are classed as coarse or fine.

Casts containing fat droplets are called fatty casts and are associated with the nephrotic syndrome (Figures 6-7 and 6-8).

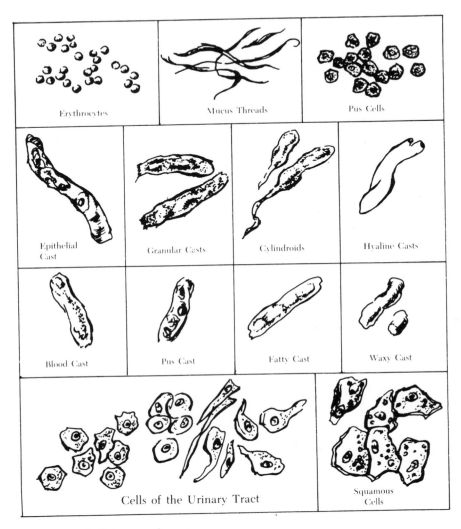

FIGURE 6-7: Urinary sediments.

For most of our purposes the routine urinalysis discussed should suffice. While there are other urine tests that may be performed, it is

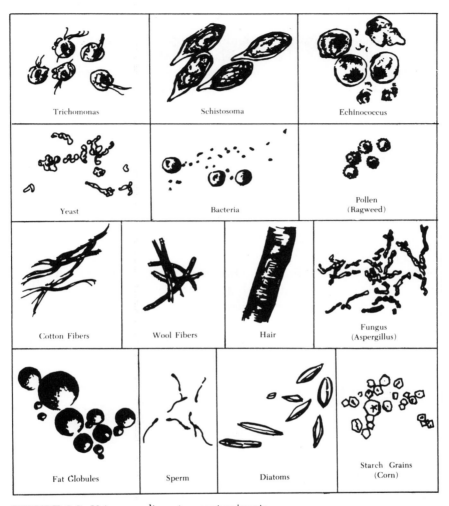

FIGURE 6-8: Urinary sediments—contaminants.

not in the scope of this text to discuss all of the possible tests. Several of the more common and important tests are described in the following.

CHROMATOGRAPHY

Chromatography is a method for the purification and/or separation of small amounts of cloudy related substances from one another. This is achieved by the slow washing, with a suitable fluid vehicle, of mixtures of the substances through an active medium. This medium differentially impedes the free movement of substances to be separated. The substances therefore travel through the medium at different rates and are thus separated.

Chromatography is used in clinical laboratories to identify sugars in urine; to separate porphyrins; for the separation and determination of urinary hydroxycorticosteroids and ketosteroids; for the separation of catecholamines and as a basis for certain commercially available and accurate tests for urea nitrogen determination, and the identification of certain bacteriological groupings.

Thin layer chromatography is chromatography but using the techniques employed in paper chromatography. This method is used in separating and identifying barbiturates and narcotics, as well as some poisons, in forensic medicine.

Gas chromatography is essentially column chromatography, employing a carrier gas to wash a vaporized sample through a column. This method has been used to separate quantitatively barbiturates and narcotics. It has been used for blood gas, and respiratory gas studies, as well as in fatty acid and steroid work.

ADDIS COUNT

The Addis Count is a centrifuged method of quantitatively estimating the formed elements in urine over a 12- or 24-hour period. The urine specimen is centrifuged and the sediment resuspended in saline. A conventional counting-chamber technique is used to record the number of leukocytes, casts, erythrocytes and epithelial cells. Normal value allows as many as 1000 casts in a 12-hour specimen, most of which are hyaline. Red blood cells rarely exceed 500,000 in the absence of disease. Various elevations in the Addis Count components occur in equally varied degrees of severity in nephritis.

ALDOSTERONE

Aldosterone is the most potent mineral-corticoid concerned primarily with renal control of electrolyte balance. It brings about an increased reabsorption of sodium chloride with increased excretion of potassium hydrogen-ion leading to a reduction of urine pH. Aldosterone also influences the blood pressure by two mechanisms: indirectly by its effect on renal retention leading to increased plasma volume, and directly by inner action with hormones of the sympathetic nervous system. Primary aldosteronism or "Conn's syndrome" is characterized by hypertension, hypokalemia, and alkaloidosis. Increased aldosterone excretion is also present in nephrotic edema, cardiac failure, decompensated hepatic cirrhosis, and secondary as well as primary aldosteronism. The secretion of aldosterone is determined by 24 hour levels in the urine. Low aldosterone level would suggest hypo-adrenalism or panhypopituitarism.

OCCULT BLOOD

Occult blood or hemoglobin in the urine is hidden blood and is referred to as hemoglobinuria. The most common cause of blood in the urine is the result of urinary calculi injuring the internal kidney and neoplasms. A hemoglobinuria may be found in disorders that are accompanied by excessive red cell destruction such as transfusion reactions, severe burns, and various chemical poisonings. During urine-specimen collection if bleeding is occurring in the urethra the first quantity of urine would contain blood. If, however, the bladder or prostate is involved then the end quantity would be bloody. If all samples collected are bloody the kidney and bladder are both involved. The most common tests performed for occult blood are the Benzidine Test, Orthotolidine Test, Guaiac Test, and the Occultest.

CALCIUM

Calcium is an inorganic cation which is present in all body fluids and in bone and teeth. There are many factors involved in the regulation of the concentration of serum calcium which is usually in a reciprocal relationship with phosphorus. The most important of these is the parathyroid hormone which is secreted when a fall in serum calcium occurs. The hormone causes 1) calcium to be mobilized from the bone by resorption, 2) calcium absorption from the intestine and the renal tubules is enhanced, 3) and phosphate secretion by the renal tubules is increased or its reabsorption by the renal tubules is inhibited. A calcium metabolism disorder may be suspected in a patient with renal calculi, bone disease, convulsions, tetany, or even complaints of malaise or fatigue. A 24 hour urine calcium test is important and should be performed after a calcium-free diet for three days. Increased values suggest hyperparathyroidism, or renal tubular acidosis. A decrease may suggest hypothyroidism, hypo-vitaminosis D, or a malabsorption syndrome.

CATECHOLAMINES

Epinephrine and norepinephrine are B-catechol ethonolamines. Normal urine contains approximately 15 percent epinephrine and 85 percent norepinephrine. Norepinephrine is constantly being secreted by sympathetic nerve endings and acts at the site of liberation to maintain vasomotor tone and blood pressure, and does not give the more general and wide-spread effects in emergency as epinephrine. Paroxysmal or persistent elevation of catecholamines in the blood or urine is diagnostic of pheochromocytoma or extramedullary chromaffin tumors. Some patients with malignant hypertension also have elevated titres. Progressive muscular dystrophy, myasthenia gravis, and drugs such as tetracycline and epinephrine may also raise the catecholamine level.

VMA

Vanillylmandelic Acid (VMA) is the urinary metabolite of both epinephrine and norepinephrine and therefore reflects the endogenous secretions of the catecholamines. It is usually wise to measure both catecholamines and vanillylmandelic acid (VMA) because one may be elevated and the other not. The measurement of VMA rather than catecholamines has gained favor because of the relatively large quantities of VMA in the urine compared to the catecholamines.

CREATINE AND CREATININE

Creatine and Creatinine are important in the physiology of muscle contraction. Creatine phosphate is the stored energy source for muscle contraction. The creatine is located intracellularly, and is not readily excreted in the urine. The creatinine is a waste product of intracellular creatine and therefore is the normally excreted compound.

Creatine in the urine is important in patients with muscle disorders; increases are found in myositis, various dystrophies, and myasthenia gravis. Urinary creatinine levels parallel serum creatinine levels and are of most importance in the evaluation of kidney function.

17-KETOSTEROIDS

17-Ketosteroids are steroids which are androgens produced in the adrenal-cortical fasciulata-reticularis, the testicular Leydig cells, and the ovary. They promote nitrogen retention, epiphysial closure, and maturation in the maintenance in male secondary sex characteristics. They may also be concerned with erotism in the female. They are bound by cortical steroid binding globulin usually bound by albumin. Abnormal elevation in 17-Ketosteroids can occur in interstitial cell tumors of the testes, female hirsutism, Cushing's syndrome, adreno-genital syndrome, adrenal cancer, adrenal adenoma, severe stress, ACTH and testosterone therapy and leutin cell tumor of the ovary. Moderate decreases occur in male eunuchoidism and castration, and severe deficiencies occur in Addison's disease, panhypopituitarism, myxedema and nephrosis.

17-HYDROXYCORTICOSTEROIDS

17-Hydroxycorticosteroids are steroids produced by the adrenal-cortical fasciulata reticularis. They are vital to all facets of metabolism and their function is to promote homeostasis. In excess they produce negative nitrogen balance, cessation of growth, wasting, thinning of the skin, osteoporosis, and reduction of lymphoid tissue. If insufficient, changes on electrolyte and water metabolism include excessive renal and extra-renal sodium loss, potassium retention, decreased serum sodium, increased serum potassium, metabolic acidosis, decreased intercellular sodium and increased intracellular potassium. There is an increase in the total body water with a decrease in glomerular filtration rate and inadequate control of blood pressure. Quantitation of 17 hydroxycorticosteroids show they are almost absent in Addison's disease and low in adrenal insufficiency, myxedema, and anterior pituitary insufficiency. There is a marked elevation in Cushing's disease, moderate in thyrotoxicosis, and a mild elevation in the first trimester of pregnancy, severe hypertension, and virilism. There may also be elevation where there is simple obesity because there is a correlation to body weight.

LACTIC DEHYDROGENASE (LDH)

Lactic dehydrogenase is the enzyme that catalyzes the reversible oxidation of lactic acid to pyruvic acid. Lactic dehydrogenase is found in all glycolyzing cells and is responsible for the formation of lactic acid in glycolysis and oxidation of lactic acid in respiration. Urinary LDH may be increased in carcinoma of the kidney, bladder, prostate, glomerulonephritis, nephrosis, renal infarction, cystitis, and in conditions which would normally show an elevation in serum LDH levels including myocardial infarction and pulmonary embolism.

PHENOSULFONPHTHALEIN (PSP)

Phenosulfonphthalein (PSP) is the dye that is injected intravenously and is eliminated by the kidneys in certain quantities at certain time periods. The test is best interpreted as reflecting the renal plasma flow or renal blood flow. The phenosulfonphthalein excretion is a proximal tubular function. An increased retention of PSP may occur in chronic nephritis, congestive heart failure, edema, and urinary tract obstruction. Increases in the excretion may be seen in hyperthyroidism, hypertension, hepatic disease, and in nephritis with increased urinary output resulting in acidosis.

PORPHYRINS

Porphyrins are related as both intermediaries and by-products in the formation of blood proteins which provide the oxygen-carrying capacity of hemoglobin, myoglobin, etc. They are normally excreted in the feces and urine in small amounts, and an increase in the different types of porphyrins may imply various pathologies. Large quantities of porphyrins in urine produce a "port-wine color." Excessive levels may occur in porphyria, hepatic disease, Hodgkin's disease, hepatic cirrhosis, and various carcinomas.

UROBILIN

Urobilin is produced from bilirubin breakdown which comes from the degradation of erythrocytes. An increase in urinary urobilin may suggest a hemolysis of hemolytic jaundice or pernicious anemia. It may also be seen in cases of infectious hepatitis, eclampsia, portal cirrhosis, congestive heart failure, malaria and lumbar pneumonia, along with certain septicemias. An increased urinary urobilin and urobilinogen in the absence of hemolytic anemias may indicate liver infection or malfunction. In liver diseases such as infectious hepatitis, obstructive jaundice, and others, bilirubin may be detected in the urine before the blood level is elevated.

CHAPTER 7
Infectious Diseases

BACTERIOLOGY

METHODS

It is essential that an adequate amount of material be obtained so that various media can be inoculated (Figure 7-1). Specimens may be examined in the laboratory by two general procedures. They may be examined by direct smear, stained or unstained, and by culture on appropriate media.

In bacteriology, the most common stain used is that of a Gram or one of its modifications. Loeffler's, methylene blue, the acid-fast stain, spore stains, capsule stains and flagella stains may be used for special purposes.

The development of techniques for conjugating antibodies with

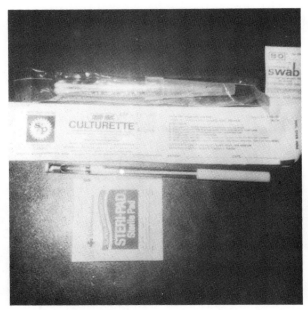

FIGURE 7-1: Three different means of specimen collection to be sent to the laboratory for culture and sensitivity studies.

fluorescein and its application to identify specific microorganisms will replace serologic methods of identifying bacteria. The fluorescent antibody or FA techniques speed up microbiologic diagnosis.

Podiatrists should inform the laboratory of the source of the specimen, the clinical problem involved, and indicate what may be suspected. If a Gram-negative organism is suspected, the specimen may be streaked directly on MacConkey's and/or Thayer-Martin's medium, or if a mycosis is suspected, Sabouraud's medium should be used.

Culture media containing whole blood is most commonly used in the laboratory (Figure 7-2). The isolation of bacteria from samples sent to the laboratory is accomplished by streaking on the surface of the blood or agar plate. The streaking is done with an inoculating loop. The purpose of streaking is to spread on inoculum so as to ensure the appearance of isolated colonies so that pure cultures can be picked for identification (Figure 7-3).

DISC SENSITIVITY TESTS

Several sensitivity tests are available and include agar dilution, tube dilution, and disc diffusion. Because of the ease of performance and flexibility of the test, the disc diffusion method has become most

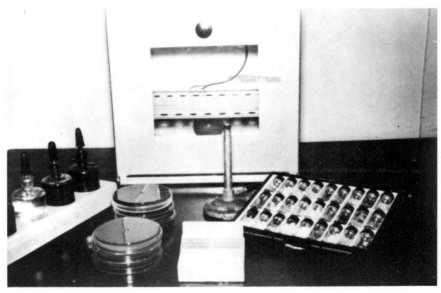

FIGURE 7-2: Small laboratory microbiology kit.

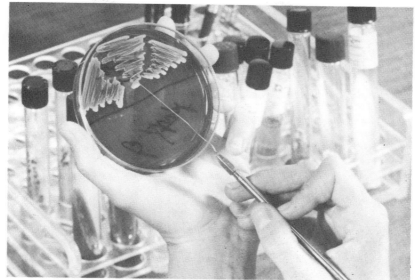

FIGURE 7-3: Inoculating cultures.

widely used. The Mueller-Hinton medium used in the plates produces rapid growth with the most commonly-encountered pathogens, contains no antibiotic inhibitors, and gives a sharp end point with the disc procedure. Many time susceptibility of the organism is determined by the Kirby-Bauer disc sensitivity test which requires overnight incubation and measurement of zones of inhibition surrounding antibiotic discs (Figure 7-4).

BLOOD CULTURES

Blood cultures are of extreme importance for the diagnosis of bacteremia and the prognosis of certain infections. Blood cultures should be obtained before antibiotics or chemotherapeutics are instituted. One simple blood culture should never be depended upon for the diagnosis of bacteremia.

In septicemia with chills, fever, or shock the pyogenic organisms can be isolated easily; when, however, the causative agent is present in only small numbers or appears only intermittently as in subacute bacterial endocarditis or brucellosis, isolation is difficult.

In drawing blood for a culture there are several principles to follow: elimination of skin organisms from the culture, elimination of air

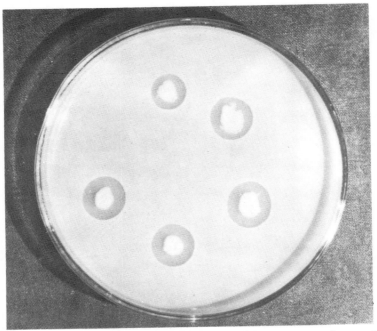

FIGURE 7-4: Disc Sensitivity Test: Note zone of inhibition surrounding antibiotic discs.

organisms from the cultures, aerobic and anaerobic culture methods should be observed, high-nutrient media should be used, and a sufficient quantity of blood is needed to ensure enough bacteria for a good growth.

ANAEROBES

Anaerobes are organisms that require a low oxidation-reduction potential which is attained by removal or exclusion of atmospheric oxygen. The importance of obligate anaerobes in infections is frequently overlooked. To most podiatrists an anaerobic infection means gas gangrene or tetanus; however, other anaerobes occur much more frequently in infections, many severe and often fatal. Among these anaerobes are bacteroides, streptococci, veillonellae, corynebacteria, micrococci and actinomycetes. In the absence of anaerobic cultures, the sample would be reported as sterile or in the case of mixed aerobic-anaerobic infections, only the organisms growing in air would be recognized.

For simplicity: any organism is considered anaerobic if, when plated on blood agar, incubated in air plus 5—10% CO_2, it appears on the anaerobic but not the aerobic plate.

The recommended method for culture is the simultaneous cultivation on anaerobic plate cultures using anaerobic jars, and in liquid media.

CLASSIFICATION

In dealing with an infection an immediate diagnosis of the nature of the infective agent is of prime importance so that appropriate antibiotic therapy may be commenced at the earliest possible moment. The first step is the Gram-staining smears which will allow a preliminary classification before final culture and sensitivity tests become available. An exact bacteriological diagnosis is necessary because microorganisms respond so differently to the various chemotherapeutic agents.

The bacteria are named and classified according to their shape, their method of staining, and the way they grow in artificial culture.

The following classification is given below along with certain diseases they cause[*]:

Classification	Disease Examples
Gram-positive pyogenic cocci	staphylococcus, streptococcus, pneumococcus
Gram-negative cocci (Neisseria)	meningococcus, gonococcus
Intestinal Gram-negative bacilli	E. coli, Bacteroides, Salmonella (typhoid, paratyphoid), Shigella (dysentery), Vibrio cholerae, Friedlander's bacillus
Corynebacteria	diphtheria
Malleomyces mallei	glanders
Mycobacteria	tuberculosis, leprosy
Spirochetes	Treponema pallidum, recurrentis
Leptospira	Ictero-hemorrhagiae, canicola

[*]From Boyd, W.: *A Textbook of Pathology*, 8th edition, Lea and Febiger, Philadelphia, 1977, p. 316, with permission.

Classification	Disease Examples
Hemophilus bacilli	He. influenzae, pertussis, ducreyi
Brucella	Undulant fever
Pasteurella.............................	tularemia, plague
Aerobic spore-bearers	anthrax
Anaerobic spore-bearers.............	Clostridia., Cl. tetani, Welchii, botulinum, Bartonella, Oroya fever

Inasmuch as the intent of this text is to focus on laboratory procedures important in podiatry, only a brief review of bacterial infections is presented.

Gram-positive Pyogenic Cocci

Staphylococci

In most hospitals staphylococci are the most common single cause of post-operative wound infections. There is an increase though in the Gram-negative bacilli including Escherichia coli, proteus, and pseudomonas.

The two species of staphylococcus that are currently identified are S. aureus and S. epidermidis or S. albus. Staphylococcus aureus is coagulase-positive and usually mannitol-positive, which means that it produces coagulase which causes clotting in human and some animal blood and it ferments mannitol. Staphylococci epidermidis is coagulase and mannitol-negative. There is a correlation between coagulase-formation and the virulence of the organism in man.

Some strains of staphylococcus aureus produce penicillinase, and are resistant to penicillin G, penicillin V and Ampicillin. Penicillinase, which is an enzyme that destroys these penicillin products, makes it necessary to use a pencillinase-resistant penicillin to subdue these infections.

Streptococci

Streptococci resemble staphylococci closely in appearance and staining character.

The hemolytic streptococci are nearly always pathogenic, whereas the non-hemolytic strains seldom cause disease.

When grown on blood agar there may be:

1. complete hemolysis, with a clear transparent zone around the colonies. This group is called beta-hemolytic streptococci.
2. incomplete or alpha-hemolysis with the production of a green pigment. This group is called Streptococcus viridans.
3. no change in the blood in the culture medium. This group is called non-hemolytic streptococci.

Streptococcus pyogens, the pus producer, belongs in Lancefield group A classification and is responsible for most cases of scarlet fever, erysipelas, puerperal sepsis, and acute tonsillitis. Rheumatic fever and glomerulonephritis are sequellae not caused by the streptococcus pyogens directly but represent an immunological response to hypersensitivity by-products.

Pneumococci

The principal disease caused by the pneumococcus is lobar pneumonia. Lesions caused by pneumococci are endocarditis, pericarditis, peritonitis, arthritis, meningitis, and infections of the nasal sinuses, etc. The total leukocyte count in pneumococcal pneumonia is elevated and there is a shift to the left in the differential count which is usual in most acute bacterial infections. The erythrocyte sedimentation rate is also increased. A leukopenia with a shift to the left is seen in severe pneumonococcal infections, especially in the presence of bacteremia.

Gram-negative Cocci

The Gram-negative cocci (the Neisseria group) include meningococcal and gonococcal infections.

Gonococcal Infections

The gonococcus, unlike the meningococcus, does not live in the body as a harmless organism. It is essentially a venereal disease, being transmitted through sexual intercourse; however, an exception would be the case in ophthalmia neonatorum. Primary cultivation of the gonococcus is difficult because of its growth requirement and its susceptibility to toxic substances often present in culture material (Figure 7-5).

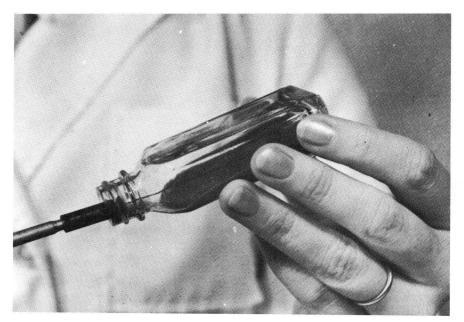

FIGURE 7-5: Gonococcus culture in transgrow media.

Carbohydrate reactions are used to differentiate gonococcus from meningococcus when positive cultures are obtained from blood, cerebral, spinal, or joint fluid. Meningococci ferment both dextrose and maltose whereas the gonococcus gives a positive reaction only with dextrose. Differentiation can also be accomplished by agglutination tests. Arthritis is a common complication but although the cocci have been isolated from the synovial fluid it is believed that the condition is allergic in character rather than a direct infection.

Differentiation of gonococcal arthritis from rheumatoid arthritis and acute rheumatic fever in many instances is very difficult. It is often impossible to culture the gonococci from the genital tract or from the joint fluid. The Gonococcal Complement Fixation Test is particularly helpful in some cases.

Meningococcal Infections

Three pathogenic possibilities open for a meningococcus to live in a human throat are:

1. A nasopharyngitis which remains localized and causes little or no discomfort.
2. There may be an invasion into the blood vessels with a set up of bacteremia without clinical disturbance or with meningo-coccemia. The Waterhouse-Friderichsen syndrome, a combination of acute meningococcemia and hemorrhage into the medulla of the adrenal glands, may completely cause destruction of both the adrenals.
3. Acute meningococcal meningitis. This suppurative meningitis may be the result of a meninogococcemia or the infection may reach the meninges from the nasopharynx by passing along the sheath of the olfactory nerves. Diagnosis is made by the examination of the cerebral spinal fluid obtained by lumbar puncture and would show a polymorphonuclear leukocytosis, increases pressure, reduced sugar content, and the presence of a meningococci which may be intracellular or extracellular.

Coliform Bacteria

Many of the coliform bacteria or Gram-negative bacilli of the in-testines are important and serve a useful purpose such as synthesizing vitamin K and members of the B complex. In addition to the useless and harmless saprophytes, some, such as E. coli and Clostridia, cause disease when implanted in tissue with diminished resistance while others, such as Salmonella and Shigella groups and the Vibrio cholerae, are dangerous pathogens which invade the intestine in con-taminated flood and water and set up violent inflammation of the wall of the bowel.

The coliform oganisms are lactose-fermenters while the majority of the pathogens are not, which is a simple means of differentiation (Figure 7-6).

Proteus and Pseudomonas

Proteus and pseudomonas are two groups of the Gram-negative motile intestinal bacilli which have come to assume increased impor-tance because of their extreme resistance to antibiotics. The proteus group ferments carbohydrates, the pseudomonas group does not, but produces distinctive pigments. Proteus vulgaris is the common species of the proteus group while the clinically important variety of

National Health Laboratories INCORPORATED

1007 ELECTRIC AVENUE
VIENNA, VIRGINIA 22180
PHONE (703) 281-5100

DR. MURRAY POLITZ
121 CONGRESSIONAL LANE
ROCKVILLE   MD 20852
                 RTE L

PATIENT NAME	SEX	AGE	ACCESSION	DATE OF ACCESSION	DATE OF REPORT	ACCOUNT NO.
DOE JOHN			247291	8/01/77	8-02-77	7081013

TEST	RESULTS		NORMAL VALUES
CULTURE & SENSITIVITY	SOURCE ABSCESS.		
HEAVY GROWTH OF STAPHYLOCOCCUS AUREUS — COAGULASE POSITIVE.			
AMPICILLIN	4+		
CEPHALOSPORINS	4+		
ERYTHROMYCIN	4+		
GENTAMICIN	4+		
KANAMYCIN	RES.		
LINCOMYCIN	4+		
CARBENICILLIN	4+		
METHICILLIN	4+		
PENICILLIN	4+		
SULFONAMIDES	RES.		
TETRACYCLINES	4+		

DAN FERIOZI, M.D. — PATHOLOGIST AND DIRECTOR

FIGURE 7-6: Culture and sensitivity report of Staphylococcus aureus in infection. (From National Health Laboratories, Inc., Vienna, Virginia, with permission.)

the pseudomonas group is Ps. aeruginosa which produces a blue-green pus. Both organisms are harmless in a healthy individual, and are harmless inhabitants of the intestines. When resistance is lowered or tissue damaged, they become dangerous invaders; proteus producing acute abscesses and pseudomonas producing thrombosis of small arteries with infarction. A bacteremia caused by pseudomonas lacks the leukocytosis and is usually accompanied by a leukopenia.

Bacteroides

Bacteroides are a group of Gram-negative, non-spore forming, non-motile, and strictly anaerobic bacilli. They are difficult to grow in culture and require enrichment with serum or even blood. They differ from the anaerobic Clostridia in not producing spores. Gas is formed in culture but not in the tissues. The definitive diagnosis of bacteroides depends on the isolation of the organisms; however the particular odor of an over-ripened Camembert cheese might suggest the possibility of an infection with this anaerobic organism.

Salmonella

Salmonella are Gram-negative, motile bacilli identical in morphologic appearance with E. coli. They are non-lactose fermenters and powerful pathogens. They are nearly all non-pyogenic in action and usually suppress the polymorphonuclear leukocytes, which usually signifies suppuration. Salmonella typhosa is the most important member of the group and causes typhoid fever which is primarily in the hemopoitic tissue and in particular the lymphoid tissue of the intestines, the abdominal lymph nodes, the spleen, and the bone marrow. The most valuable laboratory tests are:
1. Blood culture; this is most important during the first week of illness and is rarely positive after the third or fourth week.
2. The Weidel Test or Reaction which is the demonstration of the development of H and O agglutinins during the course of illness.
3. The demonstration of bacilli in the feces and in the urine.
4. The leukocyte count, which may be normal during the first two weeks; during the third and fourth weeks, however, there is usually a neutrophilic leukopenia.
During the course of the illness a normochromic anemia may develop and a proteinuria of a moderate degree is common when the fever is high.

Other Salmonella infections resemble that of typhoid but are usually milder. They would include paratyphoid, and acute gastroenteritis, or food poisoning, by the bacterial contamination of food.

Shigella

The Shigella group of bacteria which are responsible for bacillary dysentery are intestinal parasites peculiar to man. They are Gram-negative bacilli identical morphologically with coliform and Salmonella groups but are non-motile.

Dysentery is an acute colitis characterized by diarrhea. In severe cases mucus and pus are characteristically found in the stools. Blood may or may not be present.

Arthritis has been reported as a late complication in a small proportion of the cases, however, it usually occurs after the second or third week after the onset of the acute disease. The process involves the larger joints in single or multiple fashion. Usually the inflammatory condition subsides completely and spontaneously.

The laboratory diagnosis is made by the isolation and identification of the etiologic agent. Microscopic examination of the stool should always be done. The gross findings of mucus and blood may be defined by examination and the exudate of bacillary dysentery is highly cellular with a great proportion of polynuclear cells as opposed to the mononuclear exudate characteristic of protozoa infections.

Vibrio Cholerae

Vibrio cholerae is a small Gram-negative motile bacillus which causes cholera. This is an extremely acute inflammatory disease of the intestine which is caused by a powerful endotoxin produced by the organism on dying. Feces of patients with cholera may resemble rice water or starch water and contain cellular debris and masses of vibrio cholerae. In endemic areas and during periods of epidemics, cholera is easily recognized clinically. Serological identification of the organisms from the feces is usually possible and microscopic examination of the feces may reveal masses of the organisms which are often arranged linearly and in sheets. The severe fluid and electrolyte depletion in cholera is recognized by appropriate laboratory tests.

Corynebacterium Diphtheriae

The corynebacterium diphtheriae is a Gram-positive, non-motile, non-spore-forming bacillus which is characteristically club-shaped and frequently beaded in appearance. These bacilli produce an exotoxin which causes necrosis and inflammation locally and when absorbed into the blood may damage the myocardium and act on the nervous system with resulting paralysis on groups of muscles.

Diphtheria toxin is used for testing susceptibility to the Shick Test. If the subject is not immune, the toxin damages the cells of the skin and a deep red patch of inflammation develops. Children with a negative Shick Test practically never develop diphtheria. This infection usually involves the pharynx, nose, and larynx, but occasionally may occur with infection of open wounds, vulva or conjuctiva. The formation of grayish psuedo-membrane helps with the diagnosis.

Laboratory diagnosis depends upon isolation and identification of the causative organism from the lesion. A moderate leukocytosis and transient albuminuria is usually seen in all but the mildest cases.

Malleomyces

Malleomyces are organisms which are non-motile, have no capsule or spores, are Gram-negative, non-acid-fast and are relatively inert biochemically. Glanders, which is a disease of horses and donkeys and very occasionally transmitted to man, is caused by the malleomyces mallei, which is an intermediate between actinomyces and mycobacterium. Glanders is essentially a disease of equines, but grooms, veterinary surgeons, and the like may suffer from it in countries where infected animals are not destroyed. The disease, whether in animals or man, may be acute or chronic. The acute form may be an overwhelming septicemia and pyemia. The two principal features of glanders are nasal cellulitis with necrosis, and cutaneous cellulitis.

Chronic glanders is less common and takes the form of a chronic granuloma with inflammatory swelling involving the skin, lymph nodes, liver, and spleen. The diagnosis of glanders may be established by a combination of a history of exposure to horses, isolation of M. mallei, serologic and skin tests with sterile culture filtrate.

Melioidosis

Melioidosis is a rare disease caused by Malleomyces pseudomallei. This is a disease of wild rodents and some domesticated animals and characteristically is an acute febrile and fatal illness with pulmonary manifestations and occasionally undulant infection with cutaneous ulcers and visceral abscesses.

Clinical manifestations of melioidosis in man are cutaneous abscesses, diarrhea, and pneumonia. Melioidosis can be differentiated from other diseases by bacteriologic identification of the bacillus from the blood, sputum, urine or pus. An agglutination test may prove useful, but the agglutins have also been found in the serum of normal persons. The leukocyte count is often normal and the sedimentation rate usually increased. Urinalysis may show pyuria and hematuria.

Mycobacterium

The myocobacteria resist decoloration with acid after being stained intensively with hot carbolfuchsin (acid fastness) and are stained by dyes that fluoresce in ultraviolet light so that they appear as luminous rods on a dark background (fluorescent microscopy). The acid-fastness is characterisic and is usually demonstrated by the Ziehl-Neelsen technique of staining with carbolfuchsin and subsequently decolorizing with acid-alcohol. Mycobacteria retain the red color of the stain.

The tubercle bacillus resists decoloration more strongly than some of the mycobacteria which may be alcohol-fast but not strongly acid-fast. The mycobacteria consist of many saprophytic species; however, only one of the non-pathogens may deserve any mention and it is the Mycobacterium smegmatis which is often found in the smegma of both men and women. In personal discussion with Harvey Kaplan, D.P.M. of Laurel, Maryland, a case of smegma bacillus was found in a urinalysis report and almost mistaken for that of tuberculosis. The only two pathogens that are strictly parasites are those of tuberculosis and leprosy.

Tuberculosis

Tuberculosis is caused by the Mycobacterium tuberculosis. The organism grows slowly, is hard to kill, and resists drying for long periods. It neither produces an exotoxin as in diphtheria nor liberates an endotoxin on disintegrating like the typhoid bacillus. Much of its pathogenicity is related to its antigenic activity and this in turn depends on its chemical composition which is lipid, protein, and carbohydrate. Tuberculosis may be caused by two types of bacilli, human and bovine.

Today the human type is the only one of importance. Before the days of testing cows for tuberculosis and milk for pasteurization, bovine infection was extremely common. Infection with the human type is usually air-borne in patients with open pulmonary tuberculosis. This is usually due to the tiny droplets of sputum loaded with bacilli and expelled during coughing.

There are a great many clinical manifestations which may be seen in tuberculosis due to the different forms of pathologic involvement. Some of these symptoms may be generalized and others may be confined to a single anatomic organ.

A skin reaction of tuberculin may be present within five to six weeks of infection. The material used in tuberculin testing is usually a purified protein derivative and is usually applied as in the Mantoux Test, the Heaf Test, and the Tine Test. A definite diagnosis of tuberculosis depends on the demonstration by culture or animal inoculation of the mycobacterium tuberculosis.

The diagnosis of tuberculosis on purely histologic evidence is not always a simple matter. It has been pointed out that tubercle bacilli may be obtained by culture or animal inoculation from tissues on which histologic diagnosis of Hodgkin's disease and sarcoidosis has been made and conversely that a biopsy diagnosis of tuberculosis may be reversed by the bacteriologist's report of brucellosis, histoplasmosis, or coccididomycosis (Figure 7-7).

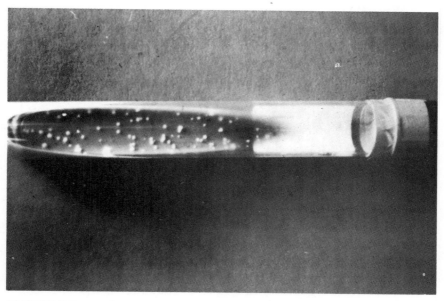

FIGURE 7-7: Mycobacterium tuberculosis on Lowensteins-Jensen medium isolated from skin lesion. (From Bionetics Research Laboratories, Kensington, Maryland, with permission.)

Leprosy

Leprosy is caused by Mycobacterium leprae which is an acid-fast organism often called Hansen's bacillus. It is more easily stained and decolorized than the tubercle bacillus. From a clinical standpoint the most important structures that are attacked are the skin, peripheral nerves and the kidneys. Disfigurement and deformity due to skin infiltration and peripheral nerve destruction in untreated patients can be extremely severe.

Two main forms of the disease are recognized: lepromatous and tuberculoid. The lepromin test corresponds to the tuberculin test for tuberculosis. A positive reaction is shown by the development of a nodule in the course of two weeks and is obtained in a normal person and in the tuberculoid while a negative result is obtained in the lepromatous form. The diagnosis can be very difficult before nodular lesions and anesthetic patches are well developed. In doubtful cases the acid-fast bacilli may be demonstrated in the discharge from the nose and the skin lesions or from a section of skin which may be removed and stained for lepra bacilli.

The standard Ziehl-Neelsen staining procedure is not sensitive enough to be used on paraffin sections of tissue if bacilli are scarce.

Spirochetes

The spirochete is a delicate spiral which is thin enough to pass through a bacterial filter. It moves actively by flagella-like structures revealed by the electron microscope. The spirochete cannot be stained with ordinary aniline dyes but in dry films it is shown by Giemsa's dark-ground illumination, the best method for fresh visualization of material.

Syphilis

Syphilis is caused by Treponema pallidum which belongs to the species of spirochetes. Syphilis, tuberculosis and leprosy all form infectious granulomata which have many features in common. T. pallidum cannot withstand drying and therefore even in a liquid environment the organism cannot survive outside the host more than a few hours. In the majority of cases, infection is acquired during sexual intercourse. It is a general systemic infection in which certain local lesions are produced. The disease is divided strictly into three stages: early syphilis, secondary syphilis, and late syphilis.

Patients suffering from syphilis are immune to reinfection. Immunity becomes established as soon as the primary lesion develops and is associated with the appearance of two distinct antibodies in the serum called syphilitic reagin and treponema-immobilization antibody. Reagin is normally present in the plasma in small amounts associated with gammaglobulin. It reacts like antibody with certain extracts of normal tissue. In syphilis, reagin is greatly increased in amount and this forms the basis of the Complement Fixation or Wassermann Test and the precipitant reaction (Kahn). The Wassermann test and the Kahn precipitation test are nonspecific tests for syphilis. The Treponema immobilization test is a specific test for a true syphilitic antibody. It is specific but requires specially designed procedures. An antigen for use in detecting the treponema antibody is available and is employed in complement fixation reactions known collectively as Reiter Protein Complement Fixation or RPCF Test. The most commonly employed test used to study a change from the serum negative to the serum positive state is the flocculation procedure known as the Venereal Disease Research Laboratories (VDRL) Test. This test is for the treponema antibodies with the three types of antigens being employed. It must be remembered that in addition to syphilis and the other Treponema infections such as Yaws, Pinta, and Bejel, there are other states not necessarily infectious which give rise on occasion to a positive reaction. The results of serologic testing that are biologic false positive reactions may approach up to 30 percent.

A positive reagin test in a person with no clinical signs or history of syphilis is significant but does not establish the presence or the diagnosis of syphilis.

Yaws

Treponema pertenue is the cause of a disease of the tropics called yaws. This infection is acquired from open sores by direct contact usually in early childhood and is non-venereal in origin. The disease also causes primary, secondary, and tertiary lesions which take the form of strawberry-like masses often occurring on the soles of the feet. In the well-developed form of this disease, the painful lesions are responsible for a peculiar, waddling, crab-like gait with the painful plantar lesions and plantar hyperkeratosis which are responsible for the peculiar waddling, crab-like gait known as "Crab Yaws."

Serologic tests similar to those used in the diagnosis of syphilis become positive and the treponema immobilization test and other specific treponemal tests also become positive and remain so for many years in untreated patients.

Relapsing Fever

Among the spirochetes of the genus Borrelia is Treponema recurrentis, the cause of relapsing fever, which is a disease found in tropical countries, although some cases have been reported in the United States. It is characterized by a recurring type of fever lasting for a few days which are separated by short periods during which the patient feels quite well. During febrile attacks the spirochetes are present in the blood in great numbers and are readily seen in a stained film, but during the afebrile intervals they vanish. The infection is conveyed by lice and ticks. Diagnosis of relapsing fever usually depends on the demonstration of Borrelia in the peripheral blood. Serologic tests are unreliable because of the confusing reactions.

Pinta

The Treponema carateum causes a disease called Pinta. It differs from syphilis in that the infection occurs through the open skin and attacks children as well as young adults. As in syphilis, three stages may be recognized. The characteristic lesion shows an increase in the number of melanophores in the dermis and increased pigmentation in the basal layer of the epidermis.

The hyperpigmented papular skin lesion gives the disease its name and when present alone may be mistaken for psoriasis or lichenified eczema.

Serologic tests for syphilis are negative during the primary stage of the disease and becomes positive soon after the appearance of the generalized lesion in the later stages.

Bejel

A non-venereal form of syphilis which is prevalent among the Bedouin Arabs is Bejel. It is a whole-community disease like measles and is acquired in childhood. The infection is contracted, usually from another child in an acute stage, probably by means of a drinking container. The earliest lesions are gray patches about the mouth followed by a papular eruption on moist areas about the body. In about a year the lesions may vanish but frequently gummata of bones, skin, and pharynx appear many years later. The Bejel Treponema is morphologically indistinguishable from Treponema pallidum and can be demonstrated from the early lesions by dark-field examination. Wassermann and Kahn tests are positive.

LEPTOSPIRA

Leptospira are much finer and more closely-wound spirals than the treponemata. There are at least 40 serologic strains which have been differentiated and have world-wide distribution but are of greater clinical importance in warm, damp, environments.

Leptospirosis icterohemorrhagiae, the cause of Weil's disease, is characterized by jaundice, oliguria, circulatory collapse, and hemorrhagic tendency. The organism is a common parasite of rats which suffer no ill effect; the kidneys, however, become infected and the leptospira excreted in the urine infect water and probably enter through cracks in the human skin. Leptospira may be identified in the blood by dark-field microscopy during the second week and reach peak titers by the third or fourth week.

The clinical laboratory findings are not unusual in the simplest forms of leptospirosis; however, in Weil's disease a polymorphonuclear leukocytosis is often seen.

HEMOPHILUS BACILLI

Hemophilus influenza is a small Gram-negative coccibacillus which requires hemoglobin for its growth. It is a common inhabitant of the nasopharynx and invades the lung and causes a secondary broncho-pneumonia. The hemophilus bacillus has played two major roles in human infections: first as a secondary invader in the influenza virus and also as a primary agent in pyogenic infections.

Hemophilus influenza may act as a primary pathogen for two tissues, the conjunctiva and meninges. It is the commonest cause of infectious conjunctivitis or "pink eye." The bacterial diagnosis may usually be obtained with the identification of hemophilus influenza or when the infection is severe by the demonstration of capsular swelling of bacteria cells found in appropriate biologic fluid. When direct examination is impossible, growth in special media may usually be obtained. In children a bacteremia is a constant feature in almost all varieties of severe hemophilus influenza and infections, and a blood culture should be specific for the disease.

CHANCROID

Hemophilus ducreyi, a Gram-negative hemophilic bacillus, is a normal parasite of the vaginal canal. The venereal disease known as chancroid is caused by the Hemophilus ducreyi. It is most common in the Orient, West Indies, and Africa. Soft chancre or chancroid is an ulcer characterized by surrounding erythema and edema but the induration of the syphilitic chancre is absent in chancroid. There are none of the sequelae which make syphilis such a serious disease. The lesions may appear on the penis and labia.

The organism cannot be cultured on ordinary media but may be cultivated by special methods from the pus if the lesion is not contaminated by secondary invaders. The typical morphology in a stained smear and typical appearance should be sufficient for a diagnosis.

PERTUSSIS

Hemophilus pertussis is a small Gram-negative hemophilic bacillus which is found in great masses in the cilia of the bronchial mucosa which causes whooping cough, also known as pertussis. This is an infectious disease of the respiratory tract in which there are spasmotic attacks of coughing with a prolonged inspiration known as a whoop. One attack of the disease confers immunity for life. There is an increase in the total leukocyte count and a definite increase in the amount of lymphocytes. The diagnosis may be made microbiologically when the Bordetella pertussis is found in great numbers. A fluorescent antibody technique is alleged the most efficient method for isolation of B. pertussis. Ordinary blood agar will not support the growth of the organism and it is necessary to make a specific request for examination of B. pertussis when a laboratory test is ordered.

BRUCELLA

The Brucella group of microorganisms are essentially pathogens of animals which may be transmitted to man. Brucellosis is the most common illness conveyed to humans from animals. The several varieties of Brucella include Br. melitensis which occurs in goats and sheep, Br. abortus which occurs in cows, and Br. suis which occurs in pigs. All three forms may infect man and may cause undulant fever.

UNDULANT FEVER

Undulant fever, known in the past as Malta fever, was originally understood to be contracted through infected goats in the Mediterranean countries, and conveyed to man through a pathogen in the goat's milk. It was later recognized that the organism was closely related to Br. abortus, the cause of contagious abortion in cattle. As the most common cause of undulant fever in man, it is responsible for eighty percent of the cases.

Infection is usually acquired through the alimentary tract by drinking unpasteurized cow's milk. The disease begins insidiously with an evening rise in temperature and the patient may be ill for some time without knowing that he has any fever. The clinical picture of the disease is varied and may consist of persistent weakness, muscle pain, low back pain, arthritis and marked perspiration with a particularly sickly-sweet odor to the sweat. These are some of the more common features which may easily go unrecognized.

A diagnosis of brucellosis can be made only on laboratory findings. The total number of leukocytes is usually normal and the differential count usually shows a relative lymphocytosis. The ESR rate may be normal or decelerated and is of little or no diagnostic value. The agglutination test with a titer of 1 in 300 or over in the presence of fever and the other clinical symptoms indicates active infection. The interpretation of lower titers is often difficult and often misleading. The brucellin skin test is similar to the tuberculin test and of no great value. A blood culture may be obtained at the height of the fever and is often negative. It has to be kept for at least a week before any growth is apparent.

PASTEURELLA

The Pasteurella are small Gram-negative, highly pleomorphic cocco-bacilli, which may take a coccal or bacillary form. Two strains are responsible for two widespread diseases in man and infections in animals. They are Pasteurella pestis, causing the bubonic plague, and Pasteurella tularensis, causing tularemia. Both of these microorganisms inhabit animal reservoirs and pass to man either directly or through the medium of insect vectors. They both produce powerful necrotizing toxins which destroy the tissue at the site of infection and are highly invasive.

TULAREMIA

Tularemia is a disease of animals which may be transmitted to man. Two types of the disease may be recognized in man and they are known as the glandular and the typhoid types.

The glandular type resembles a mild form of bubonic plague with the exception that a local lesion develops at the site of inoculation. The primary lesion and the lymph nodes undergo necrosis, suppuration, and ulceration. Bacteria have not been demonstrated in the tissue but a bacteremia occurs early and a positive blood culture can be obtained during the first week. Agglutinins appear at the end of the second week and reach their height at the end of the third week.

In the typhoid type there is no primary lesion and therefore no glandular involvement. The portal of entry is unknown but is probably unbroken skin. The disease is apt to be mistaken for typhoid fever when no primary lesion is present, or undulant fever because of a cross-agglutination; it is sometimes mistakenly diagnosed by the pathologist as tuberculosis.

The diagnosis may be confirmed by the agglutination of Pasteurella tularensis in the blood serum in the second week and also by isolation of P. tularensis from guinea pigs inoculated with material taken from the primary lesion or enlarged glands or with the patient's blood. The Erythrocyte Sedimentation Rate and C-Reactive Protein are elevated during the active stages; the leukocyte count, however, is usually normal or low. A mild albuminuria may occur during the height of the illness. Smears and cultures taken from the patient are useless.

PLAGUE

Pasteurella pestis is a small Gram-negative pleomorphic bacillus showing characteristics of bi-polar staining. It cannot exist outside the body except in the stomach of the flea. Pasteurella pestis is responsible for bubonic plague. Plague is usually caused by a vicious triangle of the rat transmitting to the flea and the flea transmitting the disease to man. Two forms of the plague are usually encountered and are bubonic and pneumonic. In the bubonic form the bacilli spread from the flea's bite to the regional axillary or inguinal lymph nodes, which become enlarged, suppurate, and form the bubos which give the disease its name.

In the pneumonic form the infection is spread by tiny droplets of sputum and although there are no bubos, the patient is over-whelmed by one of the most deadly and rapidly fatal of all infections.

The laboratory findings consist of a leukocytosis with neutro-philia in both types. There is an elevation of the ESR and other hematological tests are normal. A proteinuria and mild hematuria may accompany the acute febrile phase of the plague.

Clinical diagnosis of plague is confirmed by conventional bacteriological techniques and inoculation of susceptible laboratory animals. Examination of stained smears of bubo aspirates or sputum will usually reveal the presence of small Gram-negative bacilli.

Patients recovering from plague develop specific antibodies which may be demonstrated by the agglutination of Complement Fixation tests; these antibodies make their appearance in the second week of the disease and continue to rise in the fourth and fifth week.

AEROBIC SPOREBEARERS

ANTHRAX

Anthrax, a disease transmitted from animals to man, is prevalent in European animals especially cattle and sheep. The causative agent is Bacillus anthracis, a large, Gram-positive sporebearer. The spores are only formed outside the body and are extremely resistant and may remain a source of danger for quite some time. The infection is near-ly always conveyed through the skin, and rarely by inhaling infected material or by swallowing.

The skin lesion is the malignant pustule which starts as a pimple on the exposed part of the skin and soon develops into a vesicle con-taining clear serous or blood-stained fluid containing the anthrax bacilli. When stained with a polychrome eosin-methylene blue stain (Wright or Giemsa) the typical encapsulated bacilli will be seen. Direct cultivation of the organism should be performed on peptone agar.

ANAEROBIC SPORE BEARERS

The genus Clostridium is composed of several members which live in the soil and are readily ingested in the vegetables and establish themselves in the colon. They are strict anaerobes, and they are unable to multiply in living tissue. They confine themselves to dead tissue in which they manufacture lethal toxins. All the organisms are Gram-positive bacilli; all produce spores; and all, with the exception of Cl. welchii are motile. The spores can survive in dry earth for years and are extremely resistant to heat and antiseptics. The pathogenic members include the gas-producing anaerobes such as Cl. welchii, Cl. septicum, and Cl. oedematiens and non-gas forms including Cl. tetani, and Cl. botulinum.

GAS GANGRENE

The most common cause of gas gangrene is Cl. welchii. Gas gangrene is a disease of muscle which is at first a dull red and then becomes green or black. Bubbles or foul-smelling gas and blood-stained fluid may be pressed up and down the length of the muscle.

Gas gangrene is really a clinical and a not a bacteriologic entity and the diagnosis rests primarily on the clinical picture described, which includes pain, edema, and the general condition of the patient. It should be noted that other types of infection can cause the formation of gas in tissues, such as Klebsiella or Escherichia and may be responsible for the presence of the crepitation.

Stained smears of the exudate of wounds will give important diagnostic information if they reveal the typical Gram-positive bacilli in large numbers. It should be noted that the mere presence of Clostridia in a lesion does not mean that they are the etiologic agent in the infection because they are often found in open wounds, and may not actually participate in the cause. It is important to realize that the Clostridial infections of man are a clinical rather than a bacteriologic entity.

TETANUS

Clostridia tetani, the cause of the disease tetanus, differs entirely from the group of anaerobic gas gangrene infections. It is a muscular disorder often known as lock-jaw. The bacillus develops a terminal spore which gives a familiar drumstick appearance which can be seen in the pus from infected wounds. The growth of the bacillus is favored by the presence of aerobic bacteria and is never found in pure culture in a wound. The bacillus is a normal inhabitant in the intestines of animals and is often found in the ground. Wounds contaminated with soil or dirt from the street are always liable to infection by tetanus. It is for this reason that wounds must be protected by a prophylactic injection of the anti-tetanus serum or toxoid. As the bacilli remain in the wound they produce a powerful toxin which acts on the central nervous system.

The earliest symptom of the disease is usually spasm of the masseter muscle producing the lock-jaw effect. Because this condition is purely toxic and non-inflammatory no characteristic lesions are usually found. Symptoms are the result of an extreme hypersensitivity of the motor nervous system produced by the action of the toxin on the motor cells. As a result of this, small sensory stimuli produce a series of terrifying clonic and tonic spasms.

Bacterial examination and laboratory methods as a means of diagnosis are almost worthless. To isolate and identify Cl. tetani from a wound requires from two to three days and sometimes longer. Although Cl. tetani characteristically shows the terminal spore, other terminally-spored non-pathogenic anaerobes exist and may be present as incidental contaminants. Therefore, direct microscopic examination of wound material should be performed only by an expert. It is to be remembered that Cl. tetani can also be found among the bacterial flora on the surface of many infections without any evidence of pathogenicity. The chance of recovery of the organism on the routine biologic study does not imply that the disease will follow.

BOTULISM

Cl. botulinum is essentially a soil bacterium, but is also found in the intestines of domestic animals. It produces a disease called botulism. This member of the Clostridium differs in that the bacteria never enter the body, but produce their potent toxin in contaminated food, with resulting food poisoning.

In gas gangrene the organisms spread through the tissues they have killed by their toxins. In tetanus the organisms remain at their point of entry where they elaborate their toxin. The Cl. botulinum develop in improperly cooked food stuffs, especially those preserved in tins and stored for long periods without adequate refrigeration.

Symptoms are due to the action of toxins on the peripheral nerves. Generally within 24 hours, but sometimes within two hours after the food is eaten, the symptoms will appear. The toxins of botulism and tetanus are both strict neurotoxins differing in the site of action. The botulinus toxin acts exclusively on cholinergic nerve endings of peripheral somatic and autonomic fibers, whereas tetanus toxin acts only on nerve cells in the cerebrospinal axis.

BARTONELLA

OROYA FEVER

Bartonella bacilliformis are small minute, rod-like, motile organisms which are arthropod-borne and they are characterized clinically by an acute febrile and anemic stage known as Oroya Fever followed several weeks later by nodular cutaneous eruptions known as verruga peruviana. Both have been largely confined to Peru.

Diagnosis is usually made clinically and in the laboratory by the finding of the bartonelli in the erythrocytes in blood films in the anemic stage.

The disease is also known as Carrion's disease which if present is of the macrocytic type. The erythrocytes increase in volume and hemoglobin concentration and are hypochromic. An anisocytosis, poikilocytosis, and polychromatophilia are constantly present. Reticulocytes may constitute more than 50 percent of the erythrocytes.

RICKETTSIAL DISEASES

Although it is doubtful that podiatrists would be involved in the diagnosis or treatment of these diseases, I think a general discussion should be presented. Rickettsial diseases are caused by microorganisms which are classed between bacteria and viruses and have characteristics of both. These pleomorphic, cocco-bacillary organisms cause acute, febrile, self-limited symptoms usually accompanied by a skin rash. The group of diseases includes typhus, Rocky Mountain spotted fever, tsutsugamushi, and Q fever.

Specific serologic tests are diagnostic because after recovery from any of these diseases the blood serum contains highly specific antibodies in complement fixation or rickettsial agglutination tests. The Weil-Felix test was the only simple laboratory differentiation of these diseases for years and is still helpful in epidemics. The complement fixation test is based on a reaction of an antigen common to rickettsia and certain strains of Proteus vulgaris known as OX-12, OX-

2, OX-K. Although this test does not distinguish between groups an agglutinin titre may rise to 1:160 from a low level in diseases in the typhus and Rocky Mountain spotted fever groups.

Leukopenia is usually present except in trench fever and subsequent stages of Rocky Mountain spotted fever which also exhibits a marked anemia (Hgb 9 gm.), elevated bilirubin, and extra-renal azotemia.

PROTOZOAN INFECTIONS AND METAZOAN INFECTIONS

Protozoan and metazoan infections are parasitic infections which are common occurrences in the temperate countries. When a parasite invades a host there are four possibilities:
1. the parasite may die at once
2. it may survive without causing symptoms
3. it may survive and cause disease
4. it may kill the host.

The disease-producing parasites belong in two general groups, protozoa and worms.

Protozoa are one-celled organisms in which all functions are performed by specialized parts of the protoplasm within the single cell unit.

Metazoa are invertebrate animals made up of many cells which in aggregates are specialized into tissues and organs performing particular but coordinated functions of the entire organism.

Protozoan infections include amoebic dysentery, coccidiosis, malaria, trypanosomiasis, Leishmaniasis, toxoplasmosis, and balantidiasis.

Parasitic metazoa (Figures 7-8 to 7-11) are found primarily in the following:
A. Nemathelminthes (roundworms)
B. Platyhelminthes (flatworms)
   a. Trematoda (flukes)
   b. Cestoda (tapeworms)
C. Hirudinea (leeches)
D. Arthropoda (insects and related species).

Laboratory diagnosis would depend on each of the disease processes. Stool examination for egg larvae and the organisms itself are diagnostic. Various serologic and intradermal tests are useful but not widely available. Blood smears using special staining techniques are an aid in the diagnosis of malaria and trypanosomiasis. Visceral leishmaniasis or kala-azar is mentioned in other sections of the book as it includes enlargement of the spleen and liver, anemia, leukopenia, and hyperglobulemia.

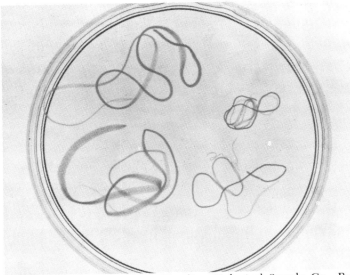

FIGURE 7-8: Roundworms. (From Carolina Biological Supply Co., Burlington, North Carolina, with permission.)

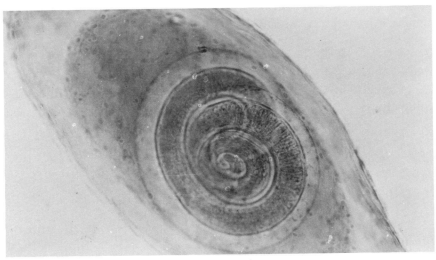

FIGURE 7-9: Pin worm (trichinella Spiralis). (From Carolina Biological Supply Co., Burlington, North Carolina, with permission.)

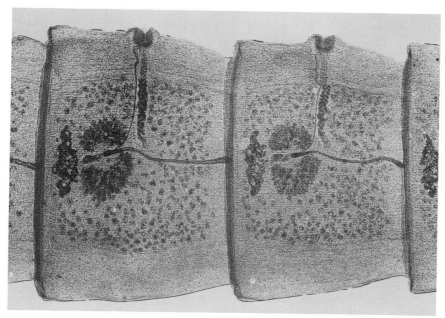

FIGURE 7-10: Taenia, W.M. (From Carolina Biological Supply Co., Burlington, North Carolina, with permission.)

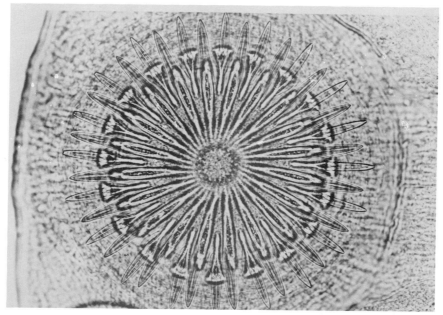

FIGURE 7-11: Taenia scolex (frontal view). (From Carolina Biological Supply Co., Burlington, North Carolina, with permission.)

VIRAL DISEASES

Viruses are the smallest and most simple biologic units that manifest the essential aspects of living substance. They are composed of an outer coat of protein and an inner case of nucleic acid. When viruses are outside cells, they appear as small particles with definite morphology. The smallest of them are no larger than the largest protein molecule and can be visualized with the electron microscope. The viruses reproduce heritable characteristics in a predictable manner during multiplication and demonstrate genetic continuity. A virus-infected cell is immune to reinfection by the virus and also immune to infection from other viruses usually related to the one which infected it

The virus-infected cell can support the reproduction of the virus which entered it and may produce new virus particles in a relatively short time.

The most common form of damage in cells supporting viral reproduction is a cytopathic effect which leads to deterioration and results in death and disintegration. Less frequent is stimulation leading to abnormal cell growth.

Bacteria are classified by their shape, and as cocci and bacilli, and by their staining properties as Gram-negative or -positive, and by their growth demands such as aerobic and anaerobic. Virus classification is more difficult and is grouped according to the target organ and similarity of action. The following classification is based on *Medical Bacterology* by Whitby and Britton as modified in *Boyd's Pathology*°:

1. The pox group including vaccinia and smallpox.
2. Neurotropic viruses including poliomyelitis, rabies, and arthropod-transmitted encephalitis including Japanese encephalitis, St. Louis encephalitis, equine encephalitis and aseptic meningitis.
3. Viscerotropic viruses such as yellow fever, infectious hepatitis and homologous serum hepatitis.
4. The herpes group including herpes simplex and other members.
5. Varicella and herpes zoster.
6. The myxoviruses group (myxo meaning mucus) which would include mumps, influenza, and Newcastle disease of chickens.

°From Whitby, L.E.H. and Hynes, M.: *Medical Bacteriology*, 6th edition, Churchill Livingstone, New York and London, 1956, with permission.

7. The lymphogranuloma psittacosis group including lympho-granuloma venereum, psittacosis, primary atypical pneumonia and trachoma.
8. Miscellanous viruses such as measles, rubella (German measles), Coxsackie viruses, adenoviruses, the common cold, warts and molluscum contagiosum.
9. Bacteriophage.

Viral infections usually produce no abnormal laboratory findings. If leukocytosis is noted, many times this is due to a bacterial complication. Viral infections may be diagnosed in the laboratory by isolation of the virus. Antibody detection in the patient's serum by neutralization, hemagglutination-inhibition or complement fixation tests are commonly used; however, a single specimen is not sufficient because of the prevalence of antibodies in the population.

See the chapter on Serologic Studies for a broader explanation of the many antibody-antigen reactions.

MYCOLOGY

CLASSIFICATIONS

Fungi are heterotropic, eukaryotic, chlorophyll-free, thallo-phyllic organisms. They reproduce by spores, which germinate into long filaments called hyphae. The hyphae grow and branch and develop into a mat of growth called the mycelium. Spores are produced from the mycelium and will germinate and form new growths. Reproduction of the pathogenic fungi is essentially asexual: the simplest type is that of the budding characteristic of yeast.

Fungi are divided into four classes: Phycomycetes, Basidomy-cetes, Ascomycetes, and Fungi Imperfecti. The majority of the pathogenic fungi belong to the latter class.

The fungi associated with human disease can be divided into those affecting only the superficial keratinized layers of the skin (dermatophytes); those affecting the deeper tissues or organs within the body (deep or systemic fungi); and those that may produce either. Techniques of isolating and identifying these organisms depend on demonstrating them in tissue by direct examination and culturing them on a media devised for that purpose.

Superficial mycoses include tinea versicolor, candidiasis, onychomycosis, tinea capitis, tinea corporis, tinea pedis, tinea cruris, peidra and trichomycosis axillaris. Systemic mycosis include actinomycosis, blastomycosis, candidiasis, chromomycosis, coccidioidomycosis, cryptococcosis, geotrichosis, histoplasmosis mycetoma, norcardiosis, sporotrichosis, aspergillosis, mucormycosis and phycomycosis (Figures 7-12 and 7-13).

LABORATORY DIAGNOSIS OF MYCOTIC INFECTIONS

The laboratory diagnosis of dermatophytosis or candidiasis depends basically on the interpretation of two tests. The first is the direct microscopic examination of scraped specimens from the involved area and the second is the culture of the specimen.

The suspected site of the fungus infection should be cleansed with alcohol to remove surface debris and the saprophytic flora. The specimen should include scrapings across the entire lesion and especially the periphery of the lesion. Nail collection may include nail and scrapings from the involved bed.

Microscopic examination includes adding a drop to two of potassium hydroxide (KOH) to the scales or scrapings from nails on a slide over which a coverslip is laid. The KOH dissolves the intercellular cementing substances reducing the keratin to a thin transparent sheet. This enables us to see the visible elements of fungi that may be present. The amount of time needed for this clearing would depend on temperature, thickness of the specimen, and concentration of the KOH. When the slide is ready, the area is scanned under low-power magnification (10 power). Fungus is seen as filaments which are

FIGURE 7-12:   FIGURE 7-13:

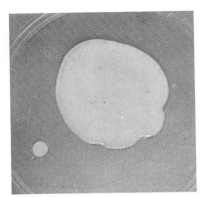

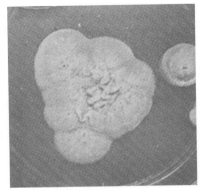

Cryptococcus neoformans.   Trichosporon cutaneum.

thread-like in appearance. These filaments if seen should then be examined under high-dry magnification (40 power). The filaments are of no particular length and may range from two-celled to multicellular structures extending across the entire field.

Arthrospores may also be seen. They are spores formed by separation of the filaments at septa. This type of filament description is seen in all species of tinea on the feet and nails and does not distinguish the different pathogens such as Tricophyton rubrum, Trichophyton mentagrophytes or Epidermophyton floccosum which are common.

Candida species can be identified by the budding filament and oval yeast cells. The arthrospores as seen in the dermatophytes are not found in Candida specimens. The filaments are thinner and more delicate appearing and pseudohyphae of elongated yeast cells joined end to end are found in Candida.

FUNGUS CULTURE

A specimen from the skin or nails is planted in the surface of a nutrient agar to grow any fungi present and to identify the species of fungus. A standard formulation for the medium should be used because of the variation in the morphology of fungi with the composition of different culture media. The medium most commonly used is similar to Sabouraud's medium with the addition of cycloheximide and antibacterial antibiotics. The isolation of dermatophytes and Candida is increased by the inhibition of saphrophytic molds and bacteria from the added substances. Recently a new medium called Dermatophyte Test Medium (DTM) was introduced and differentiates on the basis of its pH indicator, phenol red. The original yellow color changes to red as the dermatophytes cause an alkalinization of the substrate.

It is important to remember that dermatophytes are aerobic and once implanted into the culture medium they must have free access to oxygen. The cap of the vial must be kept loose after the sample is inoculated to insure a free exchange of gases. Room temperature is sufficient for growth and an incubator is not needed. Most pathogenic fungi are recognizable after two weeks of incubation. One week is too short a time for incubation and some mycologists recommend up to four weeks.

The most common pathogenic fungus isolated from the feet and toenails is Trichophyton rubrum. T. mentagrophytes, E. floccosum and Candida species account for the rest (Figures 7-14 to 7-16).

FIGURE 7-14:   FIGURE 7-15:

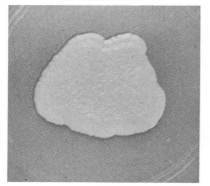   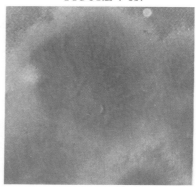

Candida albicans.   Microsporum canis.

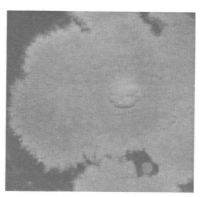

FIGURE 7-16: Microsporum gypseum.

WOOD'S LIGHT REACTIONS ON DERMATOPHYTES

Trichophyton rubrum ....light blue
T. mentagrophytes ....blue violet
T. verrucosum ....pink violet
T. tonsurans ....dark green
Microsporum audouini .... dull green
M. canis ....bright blue and pink
M. gypseum .... dull brown
Epidermophyton floccosum ....dull olive

CHAPTER 8

Disease Processes

ENDOCRINE SYSTEM

The endocrine or ductless glands are the chemical regulators of the body by virtue of the hormones which they produce. The hormones govern the processes concerned with growth, metabolism, and reproduction. It is important to note that some of the hormones control metabolism of certain inorganic elements in the body such as the adrenal cortex controlling sodium metabolism, the thyroid, iodine metabolism, and in the parathyroids, the metabolism of calcium and phosphorus. Many of the hormones are trophic in character. They may not act directly on the body cells but on another endocrine gland which may be termed the target gland. The target gland will produce its own hormones which act on the cells of the tissues and which may act at the same time to restrain the reduction of the original source of the stimuli. The brain may also play an essential part in this complex mechanism of neuro-endocrine-somatic relationship which may best be seen in the case of the pituitary. The trophic hormones may be decreased or increased in amount with corresponding changes in the hormones of the target gland. Most of the endocrine diseases are due to too much or too little hormone.

ANTERIOR PITUITARY

The anterior pituitary may be regarded as the master gland of the body. Diseases of the anterior pituitary may manifest themselves as mechanical, such as pituitary tumor, and functional, when there is deficient or excessive secretion of some or all of the several hormones secreted by the gland. The anterior pituitary produces the growth-hormone (GH) or somatotrophic hormone (STH), the adrenocortico-trophic hormone (ACTH), thyrotrophic hormone (TSH), with three gonadotrophic hormones mainly the follicular-stimulating hormone (FSH), luteinizing hormone (LH) or intestinal cell stimulating hormone (ICSH), depending on the sex, luteotropin (Prolactin), melano-cyte-stimulating hormone (MSH), and fat-mobilizing hormone.

115

The mechanisms which govern the rate at which the anterior pituitary secretes its trophic hormones depend upon the level of circulating hormones of the target glands and the action of several parts of the central nervous system, mainly the hypothalmus.

Hyperpituitarism

The main effect of hyperpituitarism is excessive growth of connective tissue and especially of the bones. The clinical result will depend on the age of the patient at which the hyperfunction becomes apparent. If it occurs in early years the result will be giantism; if at a later date it will be acromegaly, depending on whether or not ossification has been completed. The laboratory data are within normal limits.

Hypopituitarism

Pituitary insufficiency during childhood would result in dwarfism.

The hormone-induced hypopituitarism which would most commonly be encountered by podiatrists would be pituitary-adrenal suppression after prolonged administratin of adrenal corticosteroids. Corticotrophin therapy after a course of steroids is probably of little value. The patient who is being treated with corticosteroids and who faces surgery or who sustains an acute injury or infection should be treated with large doses of adrenal corticosteroids to avoid cortisone crisis.

Hypopituitarism will usually show a moderate normochromic anemia. Blood glucose concentration is often low and the serum sodium concentration will also be low.

Hyponatremia is probably related to hemodilution due to inadequate excretion of water. Urinary 17-ketosteroids and corticosteroids are decreased. The major cause of pituitary insufficiency in adult life is postpartum necrosis of the gland.

Anorexia Nervosa

Anorexia nervosa is a clinical state resulting from a psychogenic aversion to food and consequent emaciation. It has been difficult to distinguish from hypopituitarism; however, the absence of clinical or laboratory evidence of general glandular failure would help with the diagnosis.

POSTERIOR PITUITARY

The posterior pituitary or neurohypophysis produces at least two hormones, vasopressin and oxotocin. Vasopressin can produce a marked elevation in blood pressure and exerts an important anti-diuretic action on the renal tubules. This anti-diuretic hormone (ADH) increases the rate of resorption of water and electrolytes by the tubular epithelium in the loop of Henley. Oxotocin has the ability to cause contraction of smooth muscle, notably the uterus, and also acts on the contractile cells of the mammary glands, thus stimulating a flow of milk in the lactating breast.

Diabetes Insipidus

Diabetes insipidus is a clinical state resulting from a deficiency of anti-diuretic hormone (vasopressin). The lack of this hormone results in a characteristic polydipsia and polyuria with urine of low specific gravity and low chloride content. A polyuria or low specific gravity may also be frequently encountered in conditions with hyper-calcemia such as primary parathyroidism, vitamin D intoxication, sar-coidosis, and neoplastic invasion of bone. It may also be seen in states of potassium depletion such as those caused by chronic diarrhea, primary aldosteronism, and following excessive doses of deoxy-corticosterone or cortisone.

THYROID

The chief function of the thyroid gland is to maintain a higher rate of metabolism and to regulate this rate according to the needs of the body. This is accomplished by the gland's capacity to synthesize, store, and secrete thyroid hormones. The iodine-containing hormones of thyroxine and triiodothyronine are the only significant secretion products of the gland. Thyroxine is transported in the plasma in close association with protein. Triiodothyronine is less closely bound to plasma protein. The thyroid gland has a remarkable affinity for iodine and is the only organ in the body which has the power for storing that element. A test of thyroid function may include a variety of laboratory aids. Most of these tests measure different aspects of thyroid function and it is usually advantageous to run two or more of the tests when the diagnosis is in doubt. The metabolic rate is a simple and reliable index of thyroid function. In addition to hyperthyroidism, elevated values may be seen in malignant lymphoma, certain blood disorders, pheochromocytoma, asthma, congestive heart failure, and fever. Abnormally low values are seen in Addison's disease and malnutrition.

The measurement of the quantity of iodine that is precipitable with the plasma proteins is called the serum protein-bound iodine and is generally a reliable index of thyroid function. In addition to thyrotoxicosis, abnormally high values may be seen after the ingestion of large amounts of iodine, and may persist for months after administration of iodinated substances used in the visualization of gall bladder, bronchial tree, and spinal canal. In general, low serum concentrations are observed in hypothyroid states and during 24–48 hours after the administration of mercurial diuretics because of interference with the chemical analysis processes.

Tests employing radioactive iodine are widely used. The thyroidal uptake is performed after the patient is given an oral dose of I_{131} in water; however, in the laboratory a known sample of radioactive iodine I_{131} labeled as T_3 may be added to a certain amount of the patient's blood. Using the sample of blood avoids the necessity of administering radioactivity to the patient and is much more convenient as it means only obtaining a sample of blood from the patient. In circulation thyroxine is bound to a protein molecule and is referred to as thyroid-binding-globulin (TBG). A certain amount of the T_3 will combine readily with the TBG that is not already saturated with thyroxine. Interpretation of the test depends on the measurement of the remaining T_3 which is taken up by the plasma. A low uptake of small amounts of T_3 by a resin or plasma implies there are large amounts of thyroxine-deficient TBG due to a deficiency of production of the hormone. A large uptake of T_3 by the secondary plasma or resin implies that the TBG is already well-filled or saturated with ample amounts of thyroxine and that there is a condition of hyperfunctioning of the thyroid or normalcy depending upon the level.

HYPERTHYROIDISM

Hyperthyroidism or Grave's disease is a condition in which there is an excessive concentration of thyroid hormone in the blood. In patients with hyperthyroidism or thyrotoxicosis there is an elevation of the basal metabolic rate which correlates with the severity of the disease. The protein-bound iodine concentration of the serum is elevated and the uptake of radioactive iodine by the gland is increased; there is a depression in the serum concentration of cholesterol. Slight glycosuria and hyperglycemia may result. There may be negative nitrogen, calcium, and phosphorus balances and these may lead to severe dimineralization in the bones in severe cases. A hypercalcemia may be seen in 10—20 percent of the cases.

HYPOTHYROIDISM

Hypothyroidism is a condition due to insufficiency of the circulating thyroid hormone. Hypothyroid patients may be classified as having cretinism, juvenile myxedema, adult myxedema, and hypothyroidism without myxedema. These findings are determined by the duration and degree of thyroid failure and the time of life at which it occurs. Juvenile myxedema differs from cretinism in that there is no permanent retardation of mental development. In hypothyroid states the basal metabolic rate is typically low and radioactive iodine uptake is always low except in patients with metabolic cretinism or endemic cretinism when it may be normal or high. The concentration of protein-bound iodine in the serum must be low. Cholesterol concentration in the serum is about 250 mg per 100 ml. Serum TSH determination by radioimmunoassay is the most sensitive thyroid function test for the diagnosis of primary hypothyroidism and is the most reliable method of differentiating primary and secondary myxedema. An elevation in serum TSH preceeded by a reduced T_4 and T_3 is seen in primary hypothyroidism.

In secondary (pituitary) hypothyroidism there is a reduced T_4 and T_3, however, the TSH is low. In order to establish a reliable diagnosis it is essential to obtain a TSH, T_4 and a T-3 Uptake Test.

Myxedema is marked by elevations in cholesterol, uric acid, SGOT, and LDH. If tests for abnormal liver function do not yield results, thyroid dysfunction tests are indicated.

ADRENALS

The human adrenal is an organ of dual character. It consists of a cortex and medulla which are perfectly distinct in development, structure, and function. The adrenal cortex consists of three zones which produce different kinds of hormones. The outer zone, zona glomerulosa, is particularly rich in lipids, especially cholesterol. It appears to function autonomously whereas the other two zones which are the zona fasciculata and zona reticularis seem to be under the control of ACTH, the adrenocortico-hormone of the anterior pituitary. The zona fasciculata is the probable source of the 17-hydroxycorticosteroids while the zona reticularis supplies the 17-ketosteroids or androgen-like hormones.

The adrenal cortex functions in the regulation of sodium, potassium, and chloride metabolism, regulation of water balance, regulation of metabolism of carbohydrate, protein, and fat, adrogenic function, regulation of hematopoiesis and tissue reactivity, control of pigmentation, and also it has an effect on the gastrointestinal tract.

HYPOFUNCTION

Chronic adrenal cortical insufficiency is also called Addison's disease. The most definitive diagnostic procedure is the demonstration of a lack of the adrenal cortical response to the administration of pituitary corticotrophin (ACTH). In this test intravenous corticotrophin or ACTH is injected into the patient and determination of urinary 17-ketosteroids and 17-hydroxycorticoids are carried out on a 24-hour urine collection for several days. Normal patients will exhibit an increase in the excretion of these substances whereas patients with Addison's disease will show no response. Normal subjects will also respond with an eosinopenia of 80—90 percent, while Addisonian patients show little to no change in the eosinophile count.

Corticotrophin tests may also be used in conjunction with blood steroid response. Changes in blood steroid level should be observed beginning at the end of a four to eight hour infusion of corticotrophin. This method has not been accepted widely as the urine collections cannot be made.

HYPERFUNCTION

Hyperfunction of the adrenal cortex or hyperadrenocorticism may range in clinical features from Cushing's syndrome, which is an excessive adreno-cortical secretion of the 11, 17 oxygenated corticoids, hydrocortisone, and cortisone all the way to the adrenogenital syndrome which is an increased secretion of androgens from the adrenal cortex. Between these two extremes in syndromes there are many patients who present manifestations of each syndrome but to a varying degree. Hyperfunction of the adrenal cortex may also take the form of excessive production of aldosterone which is called primary aldosteronism. Cushing's syndrome, which podiatrists should be familiar with, presents a combination of severe protein depletion, typical fat distribution and a diminished carbohydrate tolerance. The urinary excretion of 17-hydroxycorticoids is increased. The level of 17-ketosteroids is lower than normal in the presence of adenoma, and normal or slightly elevated with bilateral hyperplasia. Eosinophilia, lymphopenia, neutrophilia, and polycythemia are present. Glycosuria with a diminished carbohydrate tolerance occurs frequently and occasionally diabetes mellitus may be present. In many of the cases there is a hypokalemic, hypochloremic alkalosis. The elevated resting level of urinary 17-hydroxycorticoids in the absence of an increase of 17-ketosteroids suggests pure Cushing's syndrome. The determination of urinary-free hydrocortisone which is unreduced and unconjugated is above a normal value in patients with adrenal hyperfunction.

Primary hyperaldosteronism is an excessive adrenal secretion of aldosterone which results in the syndrome of hypertension, renal wasting of potassium, hypokalemia and alkalosis. Excessive quantities of potassium are found in the urine. The serum potassium is frequently low. A normal or slightly elevated serum sodium and an elevated bicarbonate and blood pH are seen. The urine specific gravity is low and the pH is usually neutral or alkaline. The urinary 17-hydroxycorticoids and 17-ketosteroids are usually in the normal range.

PARATHYROID

The parathyroid glands are minute structures consisting of four or more in number which are difficult to demonstrate, especially as the inferior group may be embedded in the substance of the thyroid. The function of the parathyroid is to regulate the metabolism of calcium, phosphorus and bone. At a given pH there is a strong tendency for the solubility product of calcium and phosphorus to remain constant, one rising as the other falls. This constancy depends on the parathyroid hormone.

Diseases of the parathyroid gland include hyperparathyroidism and hypoparathyroidism. Renal disease may cause retention of inorganic phosphorus which tends to depress the calcium and would do so if not for the increased function of the parathyroids and subsequent hyperplasia. Just as renal lesions can influence the parathyroids so can parathyroid over-activity cause renal lesions. Hyperparathyroidism gives rise to generalized osteitis fibrosa. Pure hypoparathyroidism gives rise to tetany. Primary hyperparathyroidism may be due to single or multiple adenoma, primary hyperplasia and carcinoma. This differs from secondary hyperplasia as seen with defective calcium absorption or excessive urine loss, both frequently leading to osteomalacia with renal failure.

HYPERPARATHYROIDISM

The signs of primary hyperparathyroidism are a lower serum phosphorus, elevated serum calcium, and elevated urinary calcium. When bones become affected there is additionally an elevation of the serum alkaline phosphatase. If treatment is not instituted in cases of primary hyperparathyroidism renal failure may ensue. With renal failure the results would be a rise in serum phosphorus, a fall of serum calcium, and a fall of urinary calcium. It is important to note that a hypercalcemia is not only indicative of hyperparathyroidism. Hypercalcemia is found with vitamin D overdosage, certain bone diseases, and associated with renal damage with prolonged intake of calcium and alkali. In these cases the serum phosphatase is characteristically normal. In osteoporosis the serum alkaline phosphatase is normal.

Hypercalcemia and hypercalciuria are also found in multiple myeloma and in sarcoidosis. The serum phosphorus is normal but the serum globulin may be elevated.

HYPOPARATHYROIDISM

Hypoparathyroidism is clinically manifested as tetany. Tetany may be produced in a variety of ways, all of which are connected directly or remotely with the low calcium in the tissues. The common cause of hypoparathyroidism is the inadvertent removal of or damage to parathyroid tissue during thyroid surgery. A decrease in parathyroid hormone secretion will give rise to increase in renal tubular phosphorus reabsorption, a rise in serum phosphorus and a fall in serum calcium. As a result of the fall of serum calcium the urinary calcium falls.

PSEUDOHYPOPARATHYROIDISM

Pseudohypoparathyroidism is a condition in which the chemical abnormalities of hypoparathyroidism exist in the presence of normal or hyperplastic parathyroid glands or in the absence of renal glomerular insufficiency. It is generally part of a syndrome with developmental changes of bone. In most cases certain of the metacarpal or metatarsal bones are abnormally shortened as a result of early epiphysial union.

SYMPATHO-ADRENAL SYSTEM

PHEOCHROMOCYTOMA

Pheochromocytoma is a catecholamine-producing tumor arising from chromaffin cells of the sympatho-adrenal system. The clinical manifestations of hypertension which are usually persistent, result from the increased secretion of norepinephrine and epinephrine. The measurement of norepinephrine and epinephrine in plasma and urine provides a reliable basis for diagnosis of pheochromocytoma. A greater than two-fold elevation of plasma catecholamines is usually present during periods of hypertension. Hypertensive patients without pheochromocytoma have normal values. Fluorometric assays of catecholamines in a 24-hour urine collection usually are preferable to plasma assays for technical reasons and because elevated urinary levels are often demonstrable even during periods of non-hypertension. The measurements of urinary VMA afford an alternate and satisfactory means of diagnosis. The excretion of VMA may be elevated to at least twice the upper limit of normal.

KIDNEYS

FUNCTION

The kidneys process large amounts of water and solutes derived from extracellular fluid to produce one to two liters of urine each day. They receive from one quarter to one third of the cardiac output which means that the renal blood flow is approximately 1200 ml per minute and the renal plasma flow approximately 650 ml per minute. The tubular reabsorptive processes restore useful filtrable constituents of plasma which must be conserved in the extracellular fluid. Incomplete tubular reabsorption is responsible for the excretion of the end products of metabolism such as urea, phosphate and sulfate by the kidneys. Certain substances such as potassium, hydrogen ions, creatinine, penicillin, and certain synthetic compounds used in tests of renal function may be added to the urine by tubular secretory mechanisms.

Glomerular Filtration

In an attempt to understand the extent to which tubular reabsorption or tubular secretion participates in renal function of a specific compound we must be able to estimate the quality of the compound filtered at the glomeruli.

Clearance refers to the amount of a substance excreted in the urine per minute divided by a concentration in the plasma and this provides a measure of the glomerular filtration rate. Urea is the principle end product of nitrogen metabolism and excretion has played a very important part in the diagnosis for renal pathology. It is a diffusible compound and freely filtered by the glomeruli. The urea clearance test involves the collection of two consecutive one-hour specimens of urine and a sample of blood obtained at the mid-point of each collection. The urea clearance is usually reported as the percent of normal values. When the urine flow is 2 ml or more the urea clearance becomes maximal and can be calculated by dividing the amount of urine excreted per minute by the concentration of urea in blood. This is called the Maximal Urea Clearance. The normal is 75 ml per minute. With a urine flow of less than 2 ml per minute, the clearance may be calculated with a different method and this is called the Standard Urea Clearance. It is recommended that the Maximal Urea Clearance be used whenever possible. The Standard Clearance normal is 54 ml per minute.

In practice the blood level of urea nitrogen or BUN is often used as an index of renal function. We should note that the quantity of urea formed in the body is directly proportional to the protein intake. The quantity of urea that may be excreted by the kidneys is the product of urea clearance and the blood level of urea. As renal function declines or the protein intake increases the blood urea tends to rise until the rate of excretion equals the rate of formation. BUN normally runs 20 mg per 100 ml unless the urea clearance falls to less than 50 percent of the normal value. It is important to note that a very high protein diet or rapid cell destruction may raise the BUN to above 20 mg per 100 ml even if renal function is functioning well.

Tubular Reabsorption

The most useful constituent of plasma which is recovered by tubular reabsorption is glucose. Approximately 180 Gm of glucose are filterd daily through the tubules. Small amounts of glucose begin to appear in the urine at broad levels of 160 to 180 mg per 100 ml which is termed the renal threshold. The amount of glucose reabsorbed continues to increase until saturation of the transport mechanism is reached, which is about 300 mg per 100 ml of blood glucose.

In renal glycosuria there is a low renal threshold so that moderate amounts of glucose may escape continuously into the urine despite normal concentrations of sugar in the blood.

Tubular Secretion

Active tubular secretion is demonstrated by the fact that phenolsulfonphthalein (PSP) is excreted in the urine at a rate greater than can be accomplished by glomerular filtration. The PSP test is not a clearance procedure. It is a test of renal function which measures the amount of dye recovered in the urine at successive intervals after the injection of intravenous or intermuscular phenolsulfonphthalein.

Creatinine, the nitrogenous end produce of creatine metabolism, is excreted by a combination of glomerular filtration and tubular secretion. A greatly elevated blood creatinine usually indicates severe renal insufficiency of a chronic nature. The creatinine clearance has been used in many studies as a method of estimating the glomerular filtration rate; however, this method is only an approximation and may be an error in severe renal disease.

Water Control

The water concentration and dilution tests are performed to evaluate the capacity of the kidney to conserve or reject water. The patient is given food but no fluids for a period of twelve hours following which several successive urine samples are obtained for an estimation of specific gravity. A large amount of water is then given to the patient and the specific gravity of the urine is followed until a minimal value is reached. With the fluid restriction, the specific gravity normally rises to a level of 1.025 to 1.030; and after the water loading falls to 1.003. Patients with renal disease exhibit varying degrees of inability to concentrate or dilute the urine and may show a fixed specific gravity of values of 1.0010−1.012. In certain conditions such as diabetes insipidus there is a continued water loss in excess of electrolytes and this produces a polyuria of consistently low specific gravity. A continuous polyuria of low specific gravity is also seen in psychogenic water drinkers in whom the polyuria is a physiologic response produced by excessive fluid intake.

Electrolyte Control

Sodium

The amount of sodium excreted in the urine represents a very small fraction of that which is filtered by the glomeruli. Relatively small changes in the balance between filtration and reabsorption can produce large changes in sodium excretion. Physiologic regulation of sodium excretion usually reflects changes in both filtration and reabsorption of the kidney tubules. Aldosterone is among the best known hormones which regulate sodium excretion. In adrenal insufficiency excessive amounts of sodium are lost in the urine. This condition is tubular because it occurs even when the filtered load of sodium is reduced by a decreased filtration rate and a lowered plasma sodium. Adrenal cortical tumors which produce larger amounts of aldosterone also called primary aldosteronism will exhibit a hypernatremia. The major part of sodium which is filtered through the tubules is reabsorbed in the proximal tubule and is accompanied by chloride and bicarbonate. The bulk of sodium which passes beyond the proximal tubule is reabsorbed more distally by ion exchange mechanisms.

Potassium

Potassium renal mechanisms for regulating potassium excretion involve filtration and both tubular reabsorption and tubular secretion.

The amount of potassium excreted is about 10 percent of that filtered by the glomeruli. The capacity to reabsorb and to secrete potassium permits the kidney to vary potassium clearance from practically zero to values approaching approximately twice the rate of glomerular filtration. Potassium secretion is enhanced by potassium administration, increased intracellular concentration of potassium, cellular dehydration, hyperventilation, and other conditions which raise the urinary pH. Adrenal cortical insufficiency may decrease potassium excretion and result in hyperkalemia while adrenal cortical hyperfunction as in Cushing's syndrome and primary aldosteronism cause potassium depletion.

Potassium excretion is usually normal in severe renal disease, except in those cases in which oliguria or anuria occur.

LABORATORY DIAGNOSIS FOR DISEASES OF THE KIDNEY

Proteinuria is often the first finding noted in renal disease. Normally the quantity of protein found in urine is minimal. However, in certain disease states such as nephrotic syndrome, proteinuria may reach values of 20 gms per day or more. Orthostatic proteinuria, which is a temporary proteinuria that a person develops on assuming the erect posture without evidence of intrinsic renal disease, is believed to result in the destruction of renal venous outflow, increased venous renal pressure and increased glomerular permeability.

The examination of urinary sediment for casts, blood cells, epithelial cells, etc., is a routine procedure. Hyaline casts are formed by the intraluminal precipitation of protein in the distal portions of the nephron. Erythrocyte casts occur most commonly in acute glomerulonephritis, leukocyte casts in pyeloinephritis. Coarsely granular casts containing cellular debris are seen in advanced renal tubular disease and lipid-rich casts are found in the nephrotic syndrome.

Hematuria or erythrocytes in the urine may result from increased glomerular permeability, inflammatory processes involving the glomeruli and the urinary tract, vascular embolization, neoplasm, and similar conditions.

Chyluria is lymph in the urine. Non-parasitic chyluria is due to a rupture of a lymphatic vessel resulting in obstruction of lymphatics anywhere between the intestines and the thoraeic duct. The etiologies may include tumors, fibrosis, pregnancy, and trauma. Pyelonephritis may also be associated with this. Milky urine is the most obvious sign, but must be differentiated from pyuria and lipiduria.

Lipiduria has fat droplets which rise to the top of the urine sample after centrifugation. Lipiduria may be associated with fractures, eclampsia, diabetes, phosphorus, arsenic and carbon monoxide poisoning.

Pyuria may be due to an inflammatory process in the kidney or urinary tract. In this instance the Addis count will be elevated. The Addis count in which the formed elements of a 12-hour sample of urine are counted by a chamber-counting technique will give the number of casts, erythrocytes, leukocytes and epithelial cells that are found in the urine.

When disease processes damage large portions of the renal parenchyma most of the function tests can be expected to diminish in a more or less similar manner. Usually a few tests will indicate the presence of severe renal impairment. In the less advanced disorders in which the correct diagnosis and appropriate therapy may be of importance to the patient then the different renal function tests both for glomerular and tubular function are of greater importance.

For clinical purposes many of the simple techniques may suffice for the evaluation of renal function. Results of glomerular filtration may be obtained by measuring the clearance of urea or creatinine using the regular voided urine samples. It is important to remember that conclusions should be drawn from several samples on clearance periods performed. Usually blood levels of urea nitrogen, non-protein nitrogen, or creatinine provide a useful index of glomerular function.

Phenolsulfonphthalein (PSP) excretion is proximal tubular function. Plasma level of the PSP dye is low and its rate of excretion is determined primarily by the rate at which the dye is delivered to the tubules. Results can be interpreted as reflecting the renal plasma flow or renal blood flow. Defects in other proximal renal tubular functions such as renal glycosuria, renal aminoaciduria, and renal phosphaturia can be established by finding abnormal quantities of these materials in the urine at times when their blood levels are normal or low. Urinary acidification, ammonia excretion, potassium excretion, and the elaboration of diluted concentrating urines are functions of the more distal segments of the tubule. As in all renal function tests it should be noted that the figures obtained from a single test have limited value in the long-term prognosis for the patient. Elevations in the BUN may occur in patients with the reversible types of renal disease and patients with chronic renal disease may have virtually a zero excretion of PSP for months or years before serious complications.

LIVER

The liver is a complex vascular organ which processes the blood containing the products of digestion before it reaches the systemic cardiovascular system. The portal venous complex drains from the spleen, gastrointestinal tract, and pancreas. Diseases of the liver require a complete clinical study for appraisal because blood vessels, liver cells, and biliary drainage tracts are almost always involved in the process. As a result of this, the disease manifestations form a combination of defects in the functions of each of the three areas. The hepatic parenchymal cells not only process the blood coming from the gastrointestinal tract but also regulate the plasma composition of albumin, urea, amino acid, and glucose. In addition their function is essential in the regulation of plasma lipids, steroids, and globulin, including those involved in coagulation and transfer function. The cells adjust blood levels, respond to metabolic requirements of the body and assure biochemical homeostasis. The liver is responsible for the removal or detoxification of foreign substances and yield them readily excreted in the bile and urine or easily stored as innocuous deposits.

LIVER TESTS

The tests for liver disease are difficult to determine because complications affecting the hepatic circulation and bile flow and cellular changes arising secondarily from malnutrition, cardiovascular inadequacy, and biochemical disturbance elsewhere in the body may affect the results. It is important to discriminate between hepatocellular and biliary tract which is an excretory function.

The plasma proteins are usually effected in liver pathology with albumin low and globulin elevated. The protein electrophoretic pattern may be disturbed when tissue damage is extensive. The transaminases usually confined to the cell are released in hepatic parenchymal damage, resulting in an elevation of glutamic ox-aloacetic and glutamic pyruvic transaminase (SGOT and SGPT). Occasionally severe hepatic disease may result in a deficiency in plasma fibrinogen and prothrombin factor V and factor VII deficiency. The cephalin-cholesterol flocculation and thymol-turbidity tests are the more widely-used tests to determine changes in the plasma proteins which occur early in the onset of hepatic cellular damage. The blood non-protein nitrogen increases in advanced disease and the urea nitrogen may fall. The blood ammonia level tends to increase in hepatic failure but may be unreliable because this may occur in the interval after the blood is drawn and sent to the laboratory. The glucose-tolerance curve may show a rise in the first and second hours followed by a hypoglycemic phase. The galactose-tolerance test is of greater value because it detects impaired hepatic glycogenesis.

The excretory function may be determined by the knowledge that interference with bile flow will be followed by a retention of bilirubin, cholesterol, and bile salts. Conjugated and unconjugated bilirubin accumulate within the blood with impaired biliary excretion: conjugated in obstructive and unconjugated in hepatocellular jaundice. Parenchymal change will also result in elevated blood levels and urine output of urobilinogen.

Bromsulphthalein (BSP) is a dye that is acted upon by the liver in a manner similar to that of the transfer of bilirubin. The BSP removal test has proven useful in detecting hepatic damage that leads to impairment of biliary excretion.

The total plasma lipids, phospholipids, lipoproteins and cholesterol tend to rise to high levels during the course of biliary cirrhosis. An increase in the serum alkaline phosphatase content occurs consistently following complete and prolonged occlusion of the common bile duct.

In chlorpromazine hepatitis resulting from a hypersensitivity reaction which induces intrahepatic cholestosis, there is an elevated alkaline phosphatase and high serum bilirubin and cholesterol.

PANCREAS

The pancreas secretes a balanced electrolyte juice which adjusts the duodenal intestines to an alkaline pH for the action of the pancreatic enzymes which include alpha and beta amylase, lipase, trypsin, chymotrypsin, carboxypeptidase, leucine, amino-peptidase, deoxyribonuclease 1, ribonuclease 1, elastase, collagenase, and lecithinase.

The diagnosis of acute pancreatitis may be made by an elevated serum amylase, usually over 300 Smogyi units, with pain, tenderness, vomiting, fever, tachycardia, and leukocytosis. The serum amylase usually rises within the first 24 to 48 hours. The serum lipase usually rises later and reaches its peak in 72−96 hours. There is a leukocytosis of 10,000 to 30,000 per cu. mm with an increase in immature granulocytes. If there is bleeding into the peritoneal cavity the hematocrit and red cell count will be lowered. The blood urea nitrogen may be elevated. Hyperglycemia and occasionally glycosuria is seen. A decrease in the serum calcium is seen along with a decrease in sodium and potassium. An elevation of glutamic oxaloacetic acid transaminase, alkaline phosphatase and leucine aminopeptidase are often secondary to common bile duct obstruction or associated liver disease.

SPLEEN

The spleen is part of the hematopoietic system the principal functions of which are (1) blood formation, (2) blood destruction, (3) blood reservoir function, (4) hemolysin formation, (5) defense reaction, and (6) a hypothetical function known as hypersplenism.

The spleen is mainly involved with the production of lymphocytes and monocytes. Under certain conditions of bone marrow stress or in myelofibrosis with myeloid metaplasia, the spleen may assume the function of making all blood cells. Antibodies are also produced by the spleen. The spleen also acts as an organ of blood-cell destruction due to its unique circulation which permits stasis to occur so that phagocytosis and lytic factors can work more effectively. The spleen has been compared to a reservoir or a blood bank which can empty itself of blood when there is a sudden demand as in violent exercise, asphyxia, or hemorrhage.

HYPERSPLENISM

Hypersplenism is a term used to denote a syndrome characterized by increased destruction of normal blood cells by a malfunctioning spleen and of possible splenic inhibition of bone marrow.

In this condition there is a marked diminution in the circulating blood of erythrocytes (congenital hemolytic icterus), platelets, (thrombocytopenic purpura) and granulocytes (splenic neutropenia) or a combination of all three, termed panhematopenia. Partial to complete recovery from the cytopenia follows splenectomy. Hemolytic anemias caused primarily by accelerated red blood cell destruction in enlarged spleens may be found in several diseases such as sarcoidosis, lupus erythematosus, malignant lymphoma, chronic lymphocytic leukemia, Gaucher's disease, and myelofibrosis with myeloid metaplasia. The anemia may be moderate to severe and is usually normocytic, normochromic, or slightly macrocytic, and there are no clinical manifestations caused by the anemia with the exception of minimal jaundice. The neutropenia or thrombocytopenia associated with enlarged spleens with increased destruction of neutrophils or platelets may be seen in primary splenic neutropenia, Felty's syndrome (rheumatoid arthritis, splenomegaly and leukopenia) and kala-azar.

DISEASES OF MUSCLE

PROGRESSIVE MUSCULAR DYSTROPHY

Progressive muscular dystrophy is a hereditary disease characterized by progressive muscular wasting and weakness. The disability develops much faster in patients in whom the disease appears early in life than in those when the first symptoms appear at a later age. Pain is not usually a feature of the disease unless the contractures are fully advanced. When the onset is acute or the course rapid, with pain and tenderness, polymyositis must be ruled out. Reduction in creatinine output is seen in muscular wasting from any cause and does not differentiate muscular dystrophy from other types of wasting. However, considerable wasting does occur in muscular dystrophy and the output of creatine and the creatinine index are considerably decreased. Many times determination of urinary creatinine output will provide information on the extent of muscle wasting not readily demonstrated by other methods.

Creatinuria is also not specific for muscular dystrophy but is usually pronounced in this disease. Large amounts of creatine are excreted. Creatinuria implies a rather widespread involvement of muscles because creatine is not excreted when wasting is localized.

POLYMYOSITIS

Polymyositis is a condition which may be an acute or chronic disease of muscle characterized by reaction in both the muscle fiber and the supporting collagen connective tissue. Polymyositis may be present alone or in connection with other major systemic involvements in the group of primary myopathies or with the more generalized collagen diseases. Polymyositis has also been noted in many cases associated with malignant diseases elsewhere in the body. Muscle biopsy is useful in establishing a diagnosis but a patchy muscular involvement may be misleading and the findings in certain stages are non-specific. In many instances the muscular degeneration produces myoglobinuria and creatinuria. Exceptionally high levels of serum transaminase may be present. Blood study changes may include a leukocytosis, leukopenia, anemia, rarely an eosinophilia, elevation in the ESR and a hyperglobulinemia. Renal involvement may present with albuminuria but this is a rare finding.

POLYMYALGIA RHEUMATICA

Polymyalgia rheumatica is an illness with disseminated muscular pain and generalized symptoms usually affecting middle-aged or elderly persons. It has been regarded as a rheumatoid variant. The distal portion of the extremities are usually spared from the pain and stiffness as in many of the muscle groups. The ESR rate is elevated, a normochromic anemia, increases in serum albumin, globulin and fibrinogen are usually present. The leukocyte count is usually normal or slightly elevated.

MYOGLOBINURIA

The clinical pathologic conditions are associated with the release of myoglobin from injured muscle fibers. Myoglobin is excreted in the urine where it appears as a light or dark brown pigment which may be distinguished from hemoglobin. A myoglobinuria may induce renal damage. Myoglobin is not found in the plasma and myoglobinuria may be associated with ischemia or trauma to muscle following severe muscle exertion in normal persons and following exercise associated with hereditary absence of muscle phosphorylase. Myoglobinuria has also been found in muscular dystrophy and in instances of myositis.

ARTHRITIS

CLASSIFICATION

Arthritis or inflammation of the joint may be acute or chronic in nature. Classification for arthritis or joint disease would include:
1. Arthritis due to specific or infectious agents
2. Arthritis of rheumatic fever
3. Rheumatoid arthritis including variants such as
    a) juvenile rheumatoid arthritis (Still's disease)
    b) Ankylosing spondylitis (Marie-Strümpell disease)
    c) Psoriatic arthritis
4. Degenerative joint disease or osteoarthritis
5. Neurogenic arthropathy (Charcot joint)
6. Arthritis due to gout
7. Traumatic arthritis
8. Neoplasm of the joint.

Arthritis due to specific or infectious agents may include gonococcal arthritis, tuberculous arthritis, suppurative arthritis (usually due to streptococcus, staphylococcus or meningococcus), syphilitic arthritis, arthritis of brucellosis, typhoid fever, bacillary dysentery, rheumatic fever, rubella, and of mycotic disease to include coccidioidomycosis, histoplasmosis, blastomycosis, cryptococcosis and actinomycosis.

Before discussing the joint diseases in detail an understanding of synovial fluid, including collection and laboratory examination, is necessary.

SYNOVIAL FLUID

Synovial fluid is produced by dialysis of plasma across the synovial membrane and active secretion. The composition resembles plasma ultra-filtrate, with added hyaluronic acid. Changes in blood solute concentration require four to eight hours to affect synovial fluid levels because of slow equilibration.

Indications for aspiration of synovial fluid include arthritis of unknown etiology, possible infectious arthritis, to obtain material for culture and effusions of unknown etiology, to relieve pain or allow for increased mobility.

Aspiration must be carried out under aseptic conditions with care taken not to pass the needle through superficial or deep infection.

If enough synovial fluid is obtained because of a large amount of joint effusion, it should be divided into three or four different tubes: (1) a plain tube for gross examination, evaluation of viscosity, serologic, enzyme, and mucin clot tests, (2) a versene (EDTA) tube for cell counts and microscopic study, and (3) a heparinized tube for microbiologic studies, total protein, and glucose.

Normal synovial fluid is crystal clear and ranges from pale yellow to colorless. Turbid yellow fluid may occur with increased numbers of leukocytes in septic or nonseptic inflammation. Grossly milky fluid may occur in chronic effusion due to rheumatoid arthritis or the acute effusion of gout. Bloody fluid occurs with hemorrhagic effusions of trauma, hemophilia, or hemorrhagic villonodular synovitis. If blood is present it is important to determine whether this is due to a disease or a traumatic aspiration.

Synovial fluid in a plain tube should be examined after one hour for a fibrin clot; this would reflect damage, usually inflammation, to the synovial membrane allowing fibrinogen to enter the joint. Decreased viscosity or a poor mucin clot test suggests an alteration, destruction, or decreased production of hyaluronate due to septic or nonseptic joint inflammation.

In the mucin clot test, a large clot surrounded by clear fluid will form in a small beaker with 1 ml of synovial fluid added with 20 ml of 5 percent acetic acid.

Normal synovial fluid contains less than 200 leukocytes per cu. mm with most of these cells being lymphocytes and monocytes.

LE cells are frequently found in patients with systemic lupus erythematous (LE) and occasionally in rheumatoid arthritis (RA). RA cells are seen in 95 percent of rheumatoid joints and Reiter cells are seen in patients with Reiter's syndrome but are not specific and may be found in other joint effusions.

Cultures for suspected infectious organisms are essential but difficult to diagnose because Gram-stain and -culture are often negative. The Gram stain is one of the most widely used and important stains in bacteriology. The Gram-stain reaction is correlated with certain basic chemical and physiologic properties of bacteria and make possible the differentiation between two groups of organisms as Gram-positive and Gram-negative.

Total protein in synovial fluid averages between 1−3 grams per 100 ml. Fibrinogen is normally absent. In inflammatory joint disease, the total protein approaches that of plasma with fibrinogen present and electrophoretic patterns similar to plasma.

Synovial fluid glucose is normally 10 mg per 100 ml less than blood glucose. In nonseptic inflammatory disease processes the difference may exceed 25 mg per 100 ml.

Crystals are also important if found in synovial fluid. Monosodium urate crystals are found in almost all acute gouty joints. Calcium pyprophosphate dihydrate crystals are characteristic of pseudogout (which may mimic gout), rheumatoid arthritis, or osteoarthritis.

RHEUMATOID ARTHRITIS

Rheumatoid arthritis is a constitutional disease most characterized by a polyarthritis with a predilection for the smaller joints such as the proximal interphalangeal, the metacarpophalangeal and the metatarsophalangeal joints with the tendency for symmetrical distribution after the disease has been established. Rheumatoid arthritis is three times more common in females than in males and is usually a disease of young adults, the average age at onset being 35. Laboratory findings would include a normocytic hypochromic anemia in approximately one quarter of the patients. The serum iron is reduced but the iron-transport and iron-binding capacity of the serum are normal. The anemia is usually resistant to treatment with oral iron. A moderate leukocytosis with increase in immature cells may be present in the active cases. Urinalysis shows no characteristic changes; however, proteinuria may suggest a possibility of amyloidosis as a complication. Important in the diagnosis of rheumatoid arthritis is the test for the rheumatoid factor and also the examination of the synovial fluid. Usual flocculation tests with latex, sheep erythrocytes, or bentonite particles are positive in approximately 70 percent of adult patients with typical rheumatoid arthritis. Specific techniques including complicated inhibition techniques may be positive in 90–98 percent. The synovial fluid in rheumatoid arthritis varies from clear to turbid and frequently clots on standing. The leukocyte count may be only slightly increased in the polymorphonuclear cells. The protein content is elevated and the sugar content reduced. The mucin clot ranges from good to poor in quality and the viscosity of the joint fluid is characteristically decreased. Certain tests are nonspecific for rheumatoid arthritis and are valuable only for differentiating inflammatory arthritis from traumatic and degenerative joint disease. These tests would include the erythrocyte sedimentation rate which is elevated in nearly all patients with rheumatoid arthritis, and the C-Reactive protein which is usually positive. The serum proteins may show a decrease in albumin and an increase in globulin in severe or long standing cases; however, by the electrophoretic techniques many earlier cases show a decrease in albumin and an increase in the alpha- and gamma-globulins. Many times the gammaglobulin levels may be as high in systemic lupus erythematosus and other connective-tissue diseases. The changes in the serum proteins may be responsible for positive thymol turbidity and cephalin flocculation tests and may not be of value in the interpretation of these test results in terms of liver function. Evidence of rheumatoid arthritis may include a "Felty's syndrome" which is a combination of rheumatoid arthritis with splenomegaly and lymphadenopathy, granulocytopenia and usually anemia. The rheumatoid factor is nearly always positive and the hematologic abnormalities found are due to the hypersplenism which is explained elsewhere in this book.

STILL'S DISEASE (JUVENILE RHEUMATOID ARTHRITIS)

Certain skeletal abnormalities are seen in children because of the interference with the normal rate of growth in secondary bone centers. Tests for the rheumatoid factor are positive in a lower percentage of children with rheumatoid arthritis than in adults. However, with the more sensitive inhibition techniques used, nearly all the children will show positive results.

ARTHRITIS AGAMMAGLOBULINEMIA

Arthritis associated with agammaglobulinemia closely resembles many of the features of rheumatoid arthritis. However, the sedimentation rate is normal, other tests for the acute phase reactions are negative, and the test for the rheumatoid factor is negative.

PALINDROMIC RHEUMATISM

Palindromic rheumatism is a term that has been applied to an unusual and often recurrent form of arthritis. It consists of many attacks of acute arthritis and polyarthritis with pain, swelling, redness and disability in one or more joints. The attacks suddenly appear and develop rapidly followed by a complete remission which may be within a few hours or a day or two. There are no abnormalities in laboratory tests which have been evidenced. Differential diagnosis should include rheumatoid arthritis, gout, and systemic lupus erythematosus. There is an absence of any constitutional symptoms and the joint inflammation and discomfort subside completely between attacks. This arthritis characteristically does not respond to salicylates.

ANKYLOSING SPONDYLITIS (MARIE-STRÜMPELL DISEASE)

Ankylosing spondylitis (Marie-Strümpell disease) is a chronic disease of sacroiliac and apophysial joints and adjacent soft tissues. It is a disease of young men and the onset is the late teens or the early twenties. Less than 10 percent of these patients will show positive tests for the rheumatoid factor. The sedimentation rate may be normal in 20 percent of these patients and anemia and any abnormality in the electrophoretic pattern are not usually seen.

PSORIATIC ARTHRITIS

Psoriatic arthritis is a term used with patients with rheumatoid arthritis who also have psoriasis. The joint involvement in a majority of patients cannot be distinguished by clinical examination or radiographic findings or by histologic characteristics from rheumatoid arthritis occurring without psoriasis. It is interesting that the tests for the rheumatoid factor are rarely positive in psoriasis with arthritis.

The primary distinguishing clinical feature which may actually occur in the minority of patients with the two diseases is the inflammatory involvement of the terminal interphalangeal joint and occasionally the psoriatic involvement of the corresponding nails.

ARTHRITIS ACCOMPANYING ULCERATIVE COLITIS

Arthritis accompanying ulcerative colitis usually affects the knees and ankles. Asymmetrical involvement is more common than in rheumatoid arthritis. It may be found in 8—10 percent of patients with chronic ulcerative colitis. Tests for the rheumatoid factor are rarely positive and subcutaneous nodules are rarely seen.

REITER'S SYNDROME

Reiter's syndrome is a triad of nongonococcal urethritis, conjunctivitis and a subacute or chronic polyarthritis. The disease occurs mainly in young male adults. The main involvement may be migratory but usually is confined to a few of the larger joints after a few days. The joint usually is hot, swollen, tender with a demonstrable synovial thickening and accumulation of joint fluid. Mucocutaneous lesions may be found on the palms and soles. They appear as erythematous macules which later become hyperkeratotic waxy cones that may increase in number and form a thick keratotic crust or plaque. Laboratory findings are not diagnostic as such. A moderate leukocytosis of 10—20 thousand per cubic mm with an increase of polymorphonuclear cells is common. The erythrocyte sedimentation rate is elevated and usually correlates with the activity of arthritis. The urethral, prostatic, and conjunctival exudates along with urine, synovial fluid, and blood show no consistent pathogens when cultured. The tests for rheumatoid factors are negative and the synovial fluid changes are similar to those of mild infections or early rheumatoid arthritis.

OSTEOARTHRITIS

Degenerative joint disease or osteoarthritis is characterized by degeneration of the articular cartilage. Radiographically there is hypertrophy of the bone at the articular margins. Changes of the synovial membrane are late and minor in degree. The disease chiefly affects older persons and usually involves the weight-bearing joints. The absence of any abnormal laboratory results for inflammation or constitutional disease aids in the diagnosis. The sedimentation rate is normal and tests for the acute phase reactants are negative. The test for the rheumatoid factor is negative. The joint fluid in osteoarthritis has a low cell count ranging from a few hundred to 2—3,000 per cubic mm and the cells are predominantly mononuclear. The quantity and quality of the mucin is normal and the viscosity is not impaired.

NEOPLASM OF JOINTS

Neoplasms of joints are very rare. When there is persistent monarticular swelling without a definite traumatic history, tumor must be considered in the diagnosis. Benign soft tumors including lipoma, hemangioma, exostosis, chondroma, chondromyxoma may be suspected. Aspiration of joint fluid may sometimes be of help as in the case of the xanthomatous tumor which usually affects the knee and contains a large amount of cholesterol crystals found in the joint fluid.

DIFFERENTIAL DIAGNOSIS

The podiatrist should have great expertise in dealing with arthritic problems. Most of the diagnosis is usually dependent on the history and clinical findings. Laboratory results usually confirm the diagnosis and are not used to broadly screen the patient.

Of prime importance in the diagnosis of different arthritic problems is the rationale used by the practitioner. An excellent knowledge of the arthritic processes and a good differential diagnosis are paramount. Included in the differential diagnosis should be:

1. Hyperuricemic arthritis
2. Pseudogout—calcium pyrophosphate dihydrate crystals
3. Rheumatoid arthritis
4. Still's disease
5. Rheumatic fever
6. Psoriatic arthritis
7. Osteoarthritis
8. Lupus erythematosus
9. Traumatic arthritis
10. Sarcoidosis
11. Palindromic rheumatism
12. Intermittent hydrarthrosis
13. Fibrositis syndrome
14. Infectious arthritis
15. Gonorrheal infections
16. Syphilitic arthritis
17. Reiter's syndrome
18. Hematologic disorders such as hemophilia, leukemia
19. Synovial structure

DISEASES OF BONE

OSTEOPOROSIS

In osteoporosis there is a loss of bone mass as a result of the decreased rate of bone matrix formation. It is a disorder of the protein and mucopolysaccharide rather than of calcium and bone metabolism. This separates osteoporosis from other metabolic bone diseases in that there is no failure in the deposition of the matrix, as in osteomalacia, nor is there increased bone destruction as in osteitis fibrosa cystica. Deficiency in bone matrix formation may result from imperfect osteoblastic activity, or from the lack of or the inability to retain nitrogenous components of which the matrix is composed. Osteoporosis may be localized to the mobile parts of the skeleton or may have generalized distribution. The normal strain of activity on the skeletal system provides an essential stimulus to osteoblastic activity and when this stimulus decreases by immobilization, the effect would be a disuse atrophy of the bone. Estrogenic hormones also stimulate osteoblastic activity and a decrease in their secretion is associated with post-menopausal osteoporosis. The structural materials essential for matrix formation are inadequate under conditions of starvation, or may be diverted toward other requirements as in hyperthyroidism or in uncontrolled diabetes, with a resulting osteoporosis.

In hypovitaminosis C there is a generalized deficiency in the formation of the cement substances causing bone matrix of poor quality. If steroids are present in elevated amounts, as in Cushing's syndrome or in prolonged therapy with corticotropin and cortisone or other steroids, osteoporosis is due to the cortisone's ability to block anabolism or cause catabolism of protein tissues. Androgenic steroids have the property of producing anabolism of protein tissues; the lack of these steroids accounts for the osteoporosis seen in males with eunuchoidism and in senility.

Osteoporosis may also be seen in fragilitas ossium, acromegaly, and it may be idiopathic in nature.

In osteoporosis serum calcium, phosphorus, and alkaline phosphatase are normal. In osteomalacia phosphorus is low and alkaline phosphatase is high. In osteitis fibrosa cystica generalisata calcium is high and phosphorus low when it results from primary hyperthyroidism, the calcium is low and the phosphorus is high when it results from chronic nephritis, and the alkaline phosphatase is high from either condition. Urinary calcium may be elevated when osteoporosis is progressing. A differential diagnosis is very important and the following is presented:

1. Osteogenesis imperfecta—congenital
2. Idiopathic osteoporosis
3. Endocrine osteoporosis
   (A) Hormonal lack
      (a) Postmenopausal (estrogens)
      (b) Naturally-induced (estrogens)
      (c) Congenital ovarian agenesis (estrogen)
      (d) Eunuchoidism (androgens)
      (e) Senility (androgens)
      (f) Diabetes mellitus (insulin)
   B. Hormonal excess
      (a) Hyperthyroidism (thyroid hormone)
      (b) Acromegaly (growth hormone)
      (c) Cushing's syndrome or iatrogenic hyperadrenalism
4. Dietary osteoporosis
   A. Scurvy: inadequate intake of vitamin C
   B. Inadequate protein or calcium intake and absorption
   C. Malabsorption syndrome
      (a) Sprue
      (b) Celiac
      (c) Inflammatory disease of the digestive tract
5. Disuse osteoporosis
6. Space-flight osteoporosis resulting from reduced physical activity, increased corticosteroid release, and dietary variations.

OSTEOMALACIA

Osteomalacia is a condition where the mass of calcified bone is decreased because of a failure of calcium and phosphorus to be deposited in the matrix. It is an ability or failure due to inadequate concentration of calcium or phosphorus in the body. Osteomalacia has the same physiology as rickets except that rickets develops before epiphysial closure.

In both rickets and osteomalacia there is low blood calcium causing a compensatory increase in parathyroid activity which induces reabsorption of bone. The bone reacts with increased osteoblastic activity and raises the alkaline phosphatase. Primary hyperparathyroidism also produces the same picture. Whenever there is a low blood calcium level, due to either inadequate intake or absorption or increased urinary excretion, a rise in alkaline phosphatase occurs.

Osteomalacia may be due to:

(1) a decreased intestinal absorption of calcium which may be due to inadequate amounts of vitamin-D in the diet, excessive loss of calcium or vitamin-D through the feces, or rarely, resistance to vitamin-D.

(2) increased urinary excretion of calcium, commonly found in renal tubular acidosis, termed hypercalciuria.

(3) abnormally rapid deposition of calcium and phosphorus in the skeleton which may be seen after surgical removal of the parathyroid gland. Rarely osteomalacia may be seen in primary hyperparathyroidism; however, when this exists a very low serum phosphorus, a mild elevation of serum calcium, and a low calcium and phosphorus product may be demonstrated.

In osteomalacia a low or normal serum calcium, a low serum phosphorus, and a high serum alkaline phosphatase is seen. These findings differentiate this from the other metabolic bone diseases. Serum calcium is high in hyperparathyroidism, serum phosphorus is high in renal osteitis and serum calcium, phosphorus, and alkaline phosphatase are normal in osteoporosis. Urinary calcium is decreased when osteomalacia results from either decreased intestinal absorption or rapid deposition of calcium, and is increased when it results from renal loss of calcium.

OSTEITIS FIBROSA CYSTICA GENERALISATA

Osteitis fibrosa cystica generalisata is a condition in which the bone mass is decreased because of an increase in the rate of bone destruction. This condition is primarily seen in hyperparathyroidism and chronic nephritis. Calcium is high and serum phosphorus low in primary hyperparathyroidism whereas in chronic nephritis serum calcium is low or normal and the serum phosphorus is high. Serum alkaline phosphatase is elevated in both cases. To help differentiate this from other conditions it should be remembered that these values are normal in osteoporosis and the serum calcium is virtually never high and the serum phosphorus is almost always low in osteomalacia. The urinary calcium is high with hypercalcemia of hyperparathyroidism and is often low with glomerular insufficiency.

Osteitis fibrosa cystica disseminata, or fibrous dysplasia of bone, in which the architecture of one or more bones is distorted, presents a normal serum calcium and phosphorus.

PAGET'S DISEASE (OSTEITIS DEFORMANS)

Paget's disease is a chronic disease of the adult skeleton in which increased bone destruction, increased bone formation and abnormal architecture in newly formed bone are present. This disease is rare before the age of thirty-five and is best known for the clinical manifestation of bowing of the tibia and enlargement of the skull. The serum chemical values in Paget's disease consist of a normal serum calcium and phosphorus and an elevated serum alkaline phosphatase. The alkaline phosphatase may reach its highest levels of 100 or more Bodansky units. The initial lesion in Paget's disease is one of bone destruction and a finding of hypercalciuria might be expected with a tendency to renal stone formation and hypercalcemia. These symptoms may be found in early cases; however, when new bone formation as well as new bone destruction is increased, as generally occurs, the tendency toward calcium loss is diminished.

HYPERTROPHIC OSTEOARTHROPATHY

Hypertrophic osteoarthropathy is characterized by a syndrome which includes:
1. clubbing of the fingers
2. periosteal new bone growth involving the long bones
3. swelling and pains of the joints generally of moderate degree
4. signs of autonomic disorder such as flushing, blanching, and profuse sweating, confined mostly to the hands and feet.

When this conditin is seen it should be understood that there may be diseases found elsewhere in the body responsible for the majority of the cases such as lesions in the lungs, diseases of the cardiovascular system, diseases of the liver and diseases of the gastrointestinal tract.

Since new bone formation is the most prominent abnormality, serum alkaline phosphatase is often moderately elevated. Osteoporosis of the old bone, which may be progressive, produces decreased bone mass and increased urinary calcium. The serum phosphorus is often moderately elevated; this has not been explained. The sedimentation rate is generally elevated when arthropathy is present.

PRIMARY BONE TUMORS

Osteoblastic bone tumors such as osteogenic sarcoma, chondrosarcoma and malignant giant-cell tumor are associated with an increased alkaline phosphatase of 20−40 times normal.

Osteolytic lesions associated with bone tumors such as osteogenic sarcoma do not affect the alkaline phosphatase.

Serum calcium and phosphorus levels are normal; in massive invasions, however, the calcium level may rise and steroids are needed to bring it down.

METASTATIC BONE TUMORS

Metastatic and primary bone neoplasms may produce osteoblastic activity, thus leading to an elevated alkaline phosphatase. If the metastases are from the prostate gland, an elevated acid phosphatase may also be present.

Osteoblastic metastases may be associated with carcinoma of the breast, kidney, or thyroid, and with Hodgkin's disease. Metastic carcinomas which may produce osteolytic lesions with no rise in alkaline phosphatase levels are from the lung, rectum, kidney, and breasts.

SARCOIDOSIS

Sarcoidosis is a systemic granulomatous disease of unknown etiology. No single histologic feature may be pathognomonic for this disease or group of diseases. Along with pulmonary, cardiac, hepatic, and renal involvement, an acute polyarthritis is observed especially when erythema nodosum is present. The ankles are the most common joints involved and the arthritis will usually subside within a few weeks.

Laboratory findings are not specific for sarcoidosis but aid in the diagnosis. A leukopenia, eosinphilia and mild hypochromic microcytic anemia may be found. ESR is usually elevated along with alkaline phosphatase. Hypergammaglobulinemia is usually present and may or may not produce an elevation in total serum protein. Hypercalcemia and calciuria may be present with renal involvement. The serum phosphorus is normal or slightly elevated and helps differentiate sarcoidosis from hyperparathyroidism.

Relative tuberculin anergy is a nonspecific characteristic of the disease but the Kviem test is of great value for the specific diagnosis of sarcoidosis. In the Kviem test a patient is injected with an antigen prepared from tissues of a patient known to have sarcoidosis. After 6–8 weeks any nodule at the injection site is biopsied; histologic demonstration of an epithelioid cell granuloma is considered a positive result.

COLLAGEN DISEASES

Diseases of connective tissue, or collagen diseases, represent a group which are considered together because they have certain histologic features in common. Each of the diseases is characterized in general by systemic as well as localized features in joints, blood vessels, heart, skin, muscle, and the supporting reticulum of the internal organs.

Klinge first recognized the microscopic lesions in connective tissue as a common denominator which he described as "fibrinoid change or fibrinoid degeneration." Klemporer and his associates noted fibrinoid lesions in systemic lupus erythematosus; degeneration of the collagenous connective tissue was also noted in polyarteritis nodosa, rheumatic fever, rheumatoid arthritis, serum sickness, diffuse scleroderma, and dermatomyositis. Rich refers to these diseases as collagen-vascular diseases.

In lupus erythematosus the LE factor is present in only 70 percent of the cases; however, when the LE cell test, the fluorescent antibody test, and complement fixation are employed, 98 percent of the patients tested will react positively to one of these tests. The most characteristic antinuclear antibody is an antinucleoprotein (anti-DNP) which produces the LE cell phenomenon.

The typical LE cell consists of neutrophilic granulocyte distended by a large purple-red globular inclusion body which compresses the nucleus against the cell membrane, leaving a thin rim of

cytoplasm (Figure 8-1). In positive LE preparations polymorphonuclear leukocytes surround extracellular material which appears and
stains identical to the inclusion body forming "rosettes" (Figure 8-2).

Dermatomyositis may be characterized by a polymorphonuclear leukocytosis and, rarely, by eosinophilia. Anemia with a low
serum iron may develop. Creatinuria is in relationship to the degree
of muscle loss with myoglobinuria in severe cases. The sedimentation
rate is usually elevated. Serum transaminase enzymes are important
to follow as a guide to active myositis. Rheumatoid factor tests are
positive in a significant number of cases with LE cells rarely seen.
The serum alpha-2 and gammaglobulin may be elevated.

Polyarteritis presents a leukocytosis mainly of the polynuclear
type in 80 percent of the cases. The sedimentation rate is usually very
high and serum globulin may be increased. Anemia and eosinophilia
are noticed due to the course of the disease on various organs.

Scleroderma, in contrast to the other collagen diseases, does not
regularly present positive laboratory findings. There may be a mild
anemia and increase in sedimentation rate. The urine may contain
albumin, red blood cells, white cells, and casts.

Scleredema, a rare benign condition that follows acute infection,

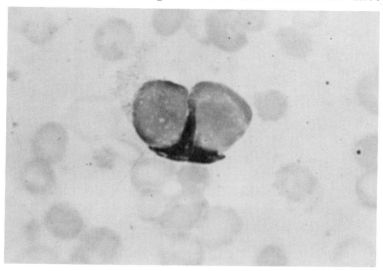

FIGURE 8-1:Lupus erythematosus (LE) cell. (From the Armed Forces Institute of
Pathology, Washington, D.C., Negative No. L-12967-43, with permission.)

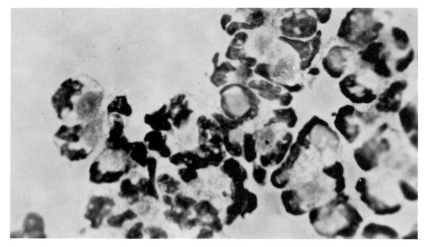

FIGURE 8-2: Cytoplasmic inclusions in aggregates of neutrophils (rosettes) as seen in lupus erythematosus. (From the Armed Forces Institute of Pathology, Washington, D.C., Negative No. L-12967-1, with permission.)

usually streptococcal, may be confused with scleroderma and dermatomyositis but involvement of the hands and feet is extremely rare.

Thrombotic thrombopenic purpura presents a thrombocytopenia of 100,000 per cu. mm or less. Renal manifestations with proteinuria and azotemia are usually present. The white cell count may be elevated and LE cells have occasionally been seen. The hemolytic anemia present is normochromic and normocytic.

ACUTE MYOCARDIAL INFARCTION

Acute myocardial infarction is the result of sudden curtailment of the myocardial blood supply. Severe and prolonged cardiac pain with other signs of cardiac damage including electrocardiographic and laboratory evidence are present.

A crushing type of chest pain or of heaviness, usually associated with a cold sweat, is often found. Nausea, vomiting, weakness, and occasionally diarrhea may accompany the pain.

It should be remembered that pain may be absent if an acute myocardial infarction occurs during an operation or in the early postoperative period when opiates are being administered.

Fever occurs in nearly all severe cases varying from 100 degrees to 102 degrees F. The temperature returns to normal by the end of the week or sooner. Leukocytosis of 12,000 to 15,000 to 20,000 is present within a few hours and disappears before the end of the week if no complications develop. The erythrocyte sedimentation rate is increased but not until after the second or third day.

The SGOT level is increased and peaks at about 24 hours, returning to normal from two to seven days. Diseases of the liver and skeletal muscle must be ruled out since the injury to these may increase the SGOT levels. The SGOT is usually not elevated in pulmonary embolism, pericarditis, or heart failure.

As an index of myocardial necrosis the LDH has greater specificity than the SGOT and is elevated for a longer duration. The increase may last from one to three weeks.

CHAPTER 9
Disorders of Metabolism

INBORN DISTURBANCES

THE GLYCOGEN STORAGE DISEASES

The "Glycogen Storage Diseases" refer to a group of inborn errors of carbohydrate metabolism characterized by excessive deposition of glycogen in tissues, associated with a deficiency of the enzymes concerned with glycogen degradation or synthesis. Six types of this group have been defined (1) hepatorenal glycogenosis (von Gierke's disease), due to lack of glucose-6-phosphatase; (2) hepatic glycogenosis (Hers' disease), due to liver phosphorylase deficiency; (3) muscle glycogenosis (McArdle's disease), due to muscle phosphorylase deficiency; (4) "limit dextrinosis" due to debrancher enzyme deficiency; (5) "amylopectinosis" due to brancher enzyme deficiency; (6) generalized glycogenosis (Pompe's disease) of unknown etiology.

The hepatorenal or hepatic glycogen storage diseases may be suspected in infants or children who have enlargement of the liver, hyperglycemia or ketosis or the development of these manifestations when food is withheld. Additional findings may be a low serum carbon dioxide, lactic acidemia, ketonuria, increased serum glycogen, and a delayed rise in blood sugar after a glucose tolerance test with low curves and rapid fall in levulose and galactose tolerance test. Hyperlipemia and hypercholesterolemia may be present and severe.

McArdle's disease is characterized by easy fatigability and muscle cramps which occur in childhood and adolescence. There may be a degree of wasting of muscles of the trunk and extremities in the third and fourth decade of life.

GALACTOSEMIA, FRUCTOSURIA, PENTOSURIA

Galactosemia, Fructosuria, and Pentosuria are all relatively rare inborn errors of metabolism characterized by excessive urinary excretion of galactose, fructose and 1-xylulose which is a pentose intermediate. A distinction should be made between these sugars and glucose so that a diagnosis of diabetes mellitus is not made in error.

RENAL GLYCOSURIA

True renal glycosuria, or renal diabetes, is an inborn metabolic defect in the renal tubular reabsorption of glucose which is characterized by a constant urinary excretion of glucose in substantial amounts in association with low or normal fasting blood sugar and normal glucose tolerance test.

True renal diabetes is relatively rare, appears early in life, and is not connected in any way with diabetes mellitus. No treatment is required as it does not interfere with normal health.

ALCAPTONURIA

Alcaptonuria is a rare disorder of metabolism of amino acids, tyrosine and phenylalanine; it is characterized by the excretion of homogentisic acid in urine. The diagnosis should be suspected early in life by diapers or linen stained black or brown by urine and by a family history of alcaptonuria.

Ochronosis is often accompanied with alcaptonuria and is a clinical state characterized by the deposition of bluish-black pigment in the cartilages, tendons, and other connective tissue. The appearance of this pigmentation, usually occurring during the second and third decades, is accompanied by degenerative changes and arthritis.

PHENYLKETONURIA

Phenylketonuria is an inborn metabolic disease of phenylalanine metabolism characterized by mental deficiency and by urinary excretion of phenylpyruvic acid and other phenyl derivatives.

Laboratory procedures are diagnostic and the demonstration of phenylpyruvic acid in the urine along with high blood phenylalanine level will confirm the diagnosis. Chromatographic and enzymatic methods are also available for diagnostic purposes.

MAPLE SYRUP URINE DISEASE

Maple syrup urine disease is characterized by the increased excretion of the branch chain amino acids leucine, isoleucine, and valine in the urine. The urine has an odor of maple syrup and there is an increase of plasma level amino acids. The disease is usually fatal in several months and treatment is unsatisfactory.

RENAL HYPOPHOSPHATEMIA

Renal tubular acidosis is characterized by a tubular defect in excretion of hydrogen ions. Azotemia due to glomerular insufficiency or tubular necrosis is not usually present in this type of disease, but is in a decline in serum inorganic phosphate concentration and a predilection towards vitamin-D-resistant rickets in children and osteomalacia in adults. In the presence of active skeletal disease the serum alkaline phosphatase is elevated. Examination of the urine for glucose and amino acid will determine whether the tubular reasorptive defect is limited to phosphate or is part of more diffuse tubular pathologies.

Renal hypophosphatemia may occur in association with other inborn defects such as renal glycosuria, amino-acid uria (Fanconi syndrome), renal tubular acidosis, and may accompany neurofibromatosis.

RENAL TUBULAR ACIDOSIS

Renal tubular acidosis is characterized by a tubular defect in excretion of hydrogen ions. Azotemia due to glomerular insufficiency or tubular necrosis is not usually present in this type of disease, but is much more common in renal acidosis associated with uremia. The excretion of alkaline or only slightly acid urine while the patient may exhibit metabolic acidosis is one of the prime diagnostic evaluations.

There may be an inability to concentrate urine and there may be a polyuria. The serum bicarbonate is reduced, the serum chloride is increased, and the serum phosphate and potassium levels are low. The serum alkaline phosphatase is increased when skeletal lesions are present.

Complications which usually appear with renal tubular acidosis include renal calculus formation, osteomalacia, and profound muscle weakness. There also may be disturbances in skeletal growth or gait pattern in the adult with spontaneous fractures occurring.

GOUT

Gout is an inborn error in metabolism characterized by hyperuricemia, by recurrent attacks of acute arthritis, and in most instances by tophaceous deposits of urate. Gouty symptoms may also be acquired as a complication of polycythemia vera and other myeloproliferative disorders.

In the diagnosis of gout, a detailed history and examination of the response of acute arthritis to colchicine are usually distinctive enough to differentiate it from the other disorders affecting joints. The demonstration of uric acid crystals in tophi, synovial tissue, or joint fluid is pathognomonic. The serum uric acid may be within normal limits in gout, but this is infrequent. In some cases, hyperurecemia may be related to renal disease with azotemia, blood dyscrasias, medications (especially diuretics) and a large number of unexplained episodes.

PORPHYRIA

Porphyria is an inborn error in porphyrin metabolism. The clinical manifestations may occur in the skin as small bulla or vesicles of the hands and the face especially after exposure to sunlight, in the nervous system as nervousness, neurasthenia or even mild hysteria, and in the abdomen as abdominal pain of a colicky nature. The examination of urine for porphobilinogen and uroporphyrin is of utmost importance. The cutaneous types are characterized by the presence of large amounts of uroporphyrin resulting in red urine. Spectroscopic examination often permits identification of uroporphyrin. If the fresh urine is normal in color the diagnosis may be overlooked unless the chromogen is looked for. If the urine is allowed to stand in the light to bring about the characteristic darkening, the uroporphyrin spectrum is then readily detected.

HEMOCHROMATOSIS

Hemochromatosis is a chronic disease characterized by the deposition of iron in the body tissues with fibrosis and functional insufficiency of those organs severely involved. The classic tetrad in hemochromatosis is skin pigmentation, liver disease, diabetes and heart failure. This iron storage disease may occur in one of three situations: (1) in idiopathic hemochromatosis, (2) in certain anemic states, (3) in long continued massive iron intake.

The most important laboratory test in the determination of hemochromatosis is the determination of plasma iron binding capacities. The excess body iron may also be identified by the intramuscular or intravenous injection of iron chelates with analysis of urinary iron.

FAMILIAL PERIODIC PARALYSIS

Familial periodic paralysis is a syndrome which is characterized by periodic attacks of flaccid paralysis which usually involve the muscles of the extremities and trunk but occasionally only affect the muscles of the arms and legs. The condition is hereditary and has its onset during the first and second decades of life. The attacks of paralysis are associated with a hypokalemia and may be precipitated by measures that may decrease the concentration of potassium in the serum.

Familial periodic paralysis must be differentiated from other disorders in which muscle weakness is associated with other disturbances in potassium. These would include primary aldosteronism, Cushing's syndrome, potassium-losing nephropathies such as renal tubular acidosis, excessive intake of diuretics, diarrheal disorders, and steroid therapy. Other muscular weaknesses are associated with a hyperkalemia which is seen in advanced renal disease, sodium depletion, and certain hereditary syndromes.

METABOLIC DISTURBANCES

ACIDOSIS AND ALKALOSIS

Many metabolic process rates are influenced by the concentration of the hydrogen ion in the body fluids. Acidosis is a condition in which the balance is disturbed to yield an increase in the concentration of the hydrogen ion, decreasing the pH. Alkalosis is a condition in which the concentration of the hydrogen ion is abnormally decreased, therefore increasing the pH value.

The system that assumes the major role in the buffering of the body fluids is the bicarbonate-carbonic acid system in the extracellular fluid.

Acid base disturbances in plasma bicarbonate concentration are primarily called metabolic acidosis and metabolic alkalosis; whereas disturbances in carbon dioxide tension are termed respiratory acidosis and respiratory alkalosis.

Metabolic acidosis arises from the addition of acid or loss of alkali from the body fluids at a rate that the normal kidney cannot maintain a normal concentration of bicarbonate in blood and extra-cellular fluid, or from kidney impairment in which acid-base balance cannot be retained with a normal addition of acid to the body fluids.

The most frequent case of metabolic acidosis is diabetic ketosis due to the production of large amounts of beta-hydroxy-butyric and acetoacetic acids.

Metabolic alkalosis, an increase in plasma bicarbonate concentration, is produced by excessive intake of alkali or abnormal loss of acid. This primarily occurs when there is sufficient dehydration to impair kidney function or when there is a depletion of body potassium, or a combination of both factors. Potassium depletion leading to hypokalemic alkalosis may arise from this continued administration of the thiazide diuretics and excess adrenal steroids.

Respiratory acidosis, an increase in carbonic acid concentration, is always the result of the increased alveolar carbon dioxide tension caused by pulmonary disease or respiratory depression from drugs or disease.

Respiratory alkalosis is produced by hyperventilation which lowers the alveolar carbon dioxide tension and carbonic acid concentration of blood.

DIABETES MELLITUS

Diabetes mellitus is a disease of carbohydrate metabolism, characterized by hyperglycemia and glycosuria and associated with a disturbance of normal insulin mechanism; it may lead to ketosis, acidosis, coma and death. So much has been written about diabetes in other texts available to podiatrists that it would be redundant to go into detailed explanation here of the disease process; it is important to realize that throughout this book there are references to the inter-relations between the many glands and conditions which affect the origin of diabetes. These would include the pancreas, pituitary, adrenals, and thyroid as well as conditions of obesity, heredity, infection, race, immunologic factors, and disturbances of the nervous system.

The elevation of cholesterol, triglycerides, and blood sugar as well as ketosis and acidosis are mentioned elsewhere in this text.

The diagnosis of diabetes may be quite simple when polyuria, polydipsia, and polyphasia are associated with an elevation of the fasting blood sugar level and with glycosuria.

The transient hyperglycemia and glycosuria occurring in other instances should not be misinterpreted as indicating diabetes mellitus. The other instances may include cerebral vascular accident, myocardial infarct, hyperthyroidism, after an injection of epinephrine, during an acute or emotional strain, in the presence of certain tumors of the adrenal medulla, severe meningitis, and in certain injuries to the brain. There may be glucose found in the urine in renal glycosuria which is mentioned earlier in this section under metabolic disturbances. Lactosuria, levulosuria, galactosuria, pentosuria, maltosuria, and alkaptonuria are rare conditions which are associated with reducing substances in the urine without elevation of blood sugar. The nature of the substances excreted should be determined in all cases of atypical glycosuria. Many of these conditions are mentioned in the text under inborn errors of metabolism.

Glucose can readily be identified by means of glucose oxidase test papers. The glucose tolerance test is useful in establishing a diagnosis of many latent diabetics; and is mentioned under the Glucose Tolerance Test.

HYPOGLYCEMIA

The condition of hypoglycemia exists when blood glucose concentration falls below 50 mg per 100 ml. There are many factors which might result in low blood glucose concentration which is basically caused from an excessive rate of removal of glucose from the blood or a decreased secretion of glucose into the blood.

The demonstration of a depressed blood sugar level is necessary to establish a diagnosis of hypoglycemia. The fasting blood glucose level may be depressed but is often normal. The Glucose Tolerance Test is useful in precipitating attacks in patients with functional hypoglycemia and they will usually develop symptoms 3–5 hours after the ingestion of glucose.

Measurement of plasma insulin concentration has been useful in distinguishing between the organic causes of hypoglycemia and functional disease.

DISORDERS OF PROTEIN METABOLISM

Agammaglobulinemia

Agammaglobulinemia is characterized by recurrent severe bacterial infections. The syndrome may have multiple etiologies and is associated with considerable impairment of antibody formation and low concentrations of plasma gammaglobulin.

There are three main types of agammaglobulinemia: transient, acquired and congenital. The infections occurring in agammaglobulinemia patients differ from those of other people by virtue of their frequency and seriousness. They are usually due to the common pyogenic bacteria.

Laboratory findings in tests on patients with agammaglobulinemia would be those signifying various acute and chronic infections. In younger patients with congenital agammaglobulinema, a neutropenia or hyperleukocytosis may accompany the pyogenic infections.

Hypoagammaglobulinemia should be suspected in patients with severe recurrent infections or in patients with thymoma or lymphoma, particularly in those with chronic lymphatic leukemia.

Multiple Myeloma

Multiple myeloma is a malignant neoplastic disease caused by proliferation of abnormal plasma cells. Multiple myeloma may present a picture of destructive bone disease along with such metabolic disease processes as diffuse renal disease, paraamyloidosis, immunological abnormality, abnormal bleeding and hyperurecemia.

In more than 90 percent of the patients an abnormal protein can be found in the serum, the urine, or both. The Bence-Jones proteinuria is demonstrated in half the cases. The use of paper electrophoresis of serum and urine protein can lead to the detection of multiple myeloma before symptoms occur. Early symptoms which may occur include unexplained anemia, elevated erythrocyte sedimentation rate, or proteinuria of unknown etilogy.

Cryoglobulinemia

Cryoglobulins are a group of serum proteins that have the common physical property of precipitating on exposure to cold and redissolving when returned to body temperatures. The clinical features of cryoglobulinemia may include a long history of cold sensitivity with skin purpura and superficial ulcers, atypical Raynaud's phenomenon, epistaxis, deafness, blotchy pigmentation of lower extremities, thrombophlebitis, retinal hemorrhage, chills and fever.

In a large percentage of patients with an elevation of the cryoglobulins many were found to have multiple myeloma, lymphogranuloma, Hodgkin's disease, subacute bacterial endocarditis, liver cirrhosis, lupus erythematosus, polycythemia vera, chronic lymphatic leukemia and kala-azar.

Cryoglobulins may precipitate other proteins, especially those involved in blood coagulation, and may therefore increase the severity of the purpura phenomenon.

Macroglobulinemia

Macroglobulinemia is characterized by symptoms of weakness, dyspnea, weight loss, bleeding tendencies and occasionally decreased visual acuity. Laboratory examinations reveal elevated sedimentation rate, hyperglobulinemia, and increased serum viscosity. An exact diagnosis can only be established by ultracentrifugation or immunoelectrophoresis of the serum and by demonstration of globulins with high molecular weight.

Amyloidosis

Amyloidosis is a disorder characterized by the deposition of amyloid in various tissues. There is no general agreement as to the best classification of the various manifestations of amyloidosis. Three main groups can be recognized: (1) generalized primary amyloidosis, (2) secondary amyloidosis, (3) localized amyloidosis. A fourth group, associated with multiple myeloma, is recognized also. Generalized secondary amyloidosis involves the parenchymatous organs such as the spleen, kidneys, liver, adrenals, lymph nodes and pancreas.

Generalized primary amyloidosis involves the mesodermal structures including the heart, tongue, larynx, skeletal muscle, kidneys, intestine and skin. Localized amyloidosis involves the mesodermal structures such as larynx, bladder, lung, oral and vaginal mucosa.

Laboratory diagnosis of amyloidosis should be kept in mind as a possible complication of any of the suppurating diseases with which secondary amyloidosis is associated.

Needle biopsy of the involved organ will help in the diagnosis. In amyloid diseases of the kidneys, the laboratory examination may reveal severe albuminuria, hypoalbuminuremia, and hypercholesterolemia. If the liver, spleen, or any of the other organs are involved, specific laboratory findings related to the organ involved would be expected.

DISORDERS OF LIPOID METABOLISM

Serum lipids are the triglycerides, phospholipids, free cholesterol, cholesterol esters, and free fatty acids. All these lipids except the free fatty acids, are present in the serum as constituents of lipoproteins. The serum lipoproteins can be fractionated by ultracentrifugation into three major fractions, each containing a characteristic lipid composition.

These lipoproteins are broken down into very low-density, low-density, and high-density fractions.

In hyperlipidemia there is an increase in the low-density lipoproteins such as cholesterol and phospholipid. They may be seen in hypercholesterolemia and secondarily in atherosclerosis, diabetes, nephrotic syndrome, and myxedema.

An increase in the very low-density lipoproteins such as the triglycerides may be seen primarily in essential hypertriglyceridemia and secondarily in severe diabetes, nephrotic syndrome, pancreatitis, acute fatty liver, von Gierke's disease, and pregnancy.

Abnormal lipoproteins may be seen primarily in biliary cirrhosis and biliary obstruction from all causes including hepatitis.

A condition of hypolipidemia shows a decrease in low-density lipoproteins such as cholesterol; this may be seen primarily in acanthocytosis and secondarily in starvation and malabsorption syndromes. There may be a decrease in the high-density lipoproteins which is seen primarily in Tangier disease and secondarily in liver disease.

Production of xanthomas in essential hypercholesterolemia and essential hypertriglyceridemia should be noticed by the podiatrist. The appearance of these lesions should suggest a disorder of lipid metabolism and it would be wise to order a cholesterol and triglyceride level to help establish a diagnosis.

CHAPTER 10

Pathological Significance of Chemistry Tests

AUTOMATION

Most large laboratories and hospital laboratories run their tests by automated procedures which save time and money due to the increasing number of tests being performed. The Auto-analyzer® ° utilizes a continuous-flow system, each operation being automatically performed as the stream of specimen liquid is propelled through the system. A long channel runs from the specimen pick up through the detecting module. The reaction procedures performed include heating, incubation, digestion, isolation, and separation as the specimen flows through modular units. By measuring the optical density of a reagent stream, a baseline is established with each sample being recorded as a peak. In the usual laboratory techniques, reactions are brought to completion and final volumes are measured (Figure 10-1). In the Auto-analyzer® ratios are used, and it is not

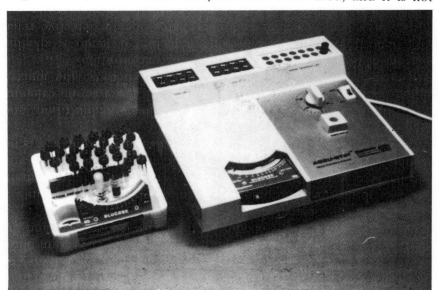

FIGURE 10-1: Clay-Adams Accu-Stat® ° ° machine for office chemistries.

°Technicon Instruments Corp., Tarrytown, New York
° °Clay-Adams Co., New York, New York

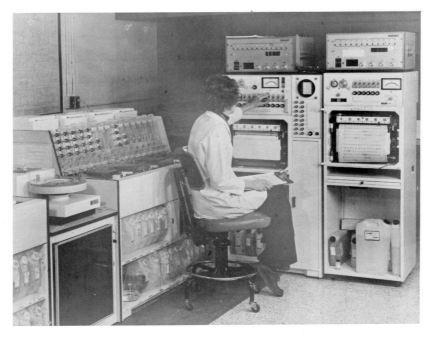

FIGURE 10-2: Technicon SMA Auto-analyzer® System. (From Technicon Instruments Corp., Tarrytown, New York, with permission.)

necessary for reactions to be carried to completion (Figures 10-2 and 10-3).

ACETONE

Acetone or ketone bodies are comprised of acetoacetate, beta-hydroxybutyrate and acetone, intermediates in the metabolic oxidation of fat. They accumulate in the blood and are excreted in the urine when glucose metabolism is impaired resulting in acidosis. Diabetes mellitus and starvation are typical situations in which ketone bodies are increased.

ALBUMIN

Albumin is produced in the liver and makes up the largest percentage (45–55%) of the total blood proteins (6 to 8 grams per

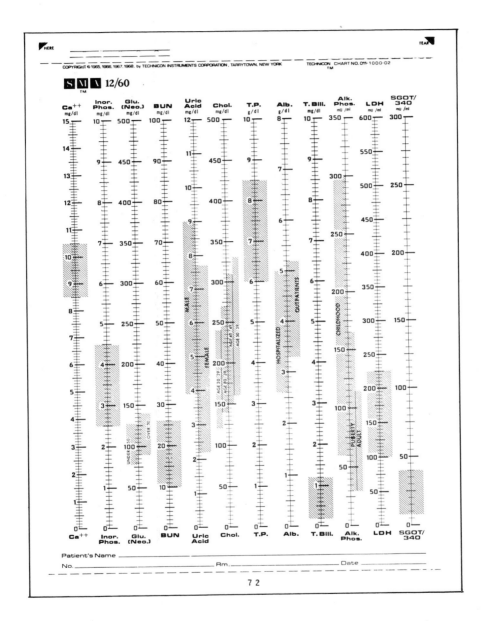

FIGURE 10-3: Serum Chemistry graph from SMA 12/60®. (From Technicon Instruments Corp., Tarrytown, New York, with permission.)

100 milliliters). Albumin is largely responsible for the colloid osomtic pressure between blood and tissue fluids. Serum albumin levels are rarely increased. Liver disease is the usual cause of a reduction which in turn disturbs the osmotic pressure in the body, resulting in fluid transfer and edema.

It takes approximately two to three weeks to deplete albumin and therefore acute liver disease may not immediately affect the serum albumin level. Other causes of a reduced albumin level include the malabsorption syndrome, nephrosis, congestive heart failure, eclampsia, poor nutrition, starvation, and excess intravenous fluids.

ALDOLASE

Aldolase is a glycolytic enzyme which catalyzes the reversible splitting of fructose-1, 6-diphosphate to form one molecule of dihydrozyacetone phosphate and glyceraldelyde 3-phospate. Aldolase may be markedly elevated in progressive muscular dystrophy, and slightly elevated in myocardial infarction, hepatitis and carcinoma of the prostate.

ALDOSTERONE

Aldosterone is the most potent mineralo-corticoid concerned primarily with renal control of electrolyte balance. It brings about an increased reabsorption of sodium and chloride with an increased excretion of potassium and hydrogen ion, leading to a reduction of urine pH. Aldosterone also influences blood pressure by two mechanisms: indirectly by its effect on renal retention of sodium leading to increased plasma volume, and directly by an interaction with hormones of the sympathetic nervous system. Primary aldosteronism or Conn's syndrome is characterized by hypertension, hypokalemia, and alkalosis. Increased aldosterone excretion is also present in nephrotic edema, cardiac failure, decompensated hepatic cirrhosis, and secondary as well as primary aldosteronism.

A/G RATIO (SERUM PROTEIN FRACTIONATION)

The albumin and globulin fractions of serum often become altered in disease. The albumin, when altered quantitively, is almost always low, while the globulin tends to increase. Usually the total protein is lowered as a result. Whatever the magnitude of alteration, the two fractions tend to balance each other and therefore diminish the clinical inferences which may be suspected from a total protein alone. Information regarding the relative serum concentration of albumin and globulin are considerably more important.

BLOOD AMMONIA-ENDOGENOUS AMMONIA

Blood ammonia-endogenous ammonia results from deaminization of protein and other amino compounds during metabolism. It is detoxified by the liver into urea. It is clinically significant in the differential diagnosis of stupor and coma, in cases of cirrhosis, and in the determination of the patency of portacaval shunts.

AMYLASE

Amylases, enzymes which catalyze the hydrolysis of starch, are of two types: alpha and beta amylase. They are produced primarily by the pancreas and salivary glands. An abnormal elevation, up to 30 to 40 times normal, is noted in acute pancreatitis. Moderate elevations are seen in chronic pancreatitis, mumps, renal insufficiency, cancer of the pancreas, and acute biliary obstruction due to common duct stone. Hepatobiliary disease is characterized by low serum amylase levels.

ARSENIC

Arsenic poisoning is mentioned only because ingestion of rat poisoning, insecticides, and especially paint are the usual causes and the chronic symptoms may be noticed by podiatrists. The chronic symptoms include fatigue, skin pigmentation, exfoliative dermatitis, paralysis and atrophy of muscles, sensory and visual disturbances. In serum nearly all is protein-bound and it is widely distributed in all soft tissue organs, especially the keratinous structures, hair, skin, and nails.

BILIRUBIN

Bilirubin arises from degraduation of red blood cells, is conjugated in the liver, and secreted through the bile ducts into the duodenum. Clinical jaundice refers to yellowing of various tissues associated with hyperbilirubinemia. There are basically two forms of jaundice: (1) retention jaundice of hemolytic or nonhemolytic organ; (2) regurgitation jaundice from either medical extrahepatic obstruction or parenchymatous extrahepatic obstruction resulting from pathological change in liver cells.

BROMSULFOPHTHALEIN EXCRETION TEST (BSP)

The indicator dye is given intravenously and by examination of the patient's serum after a time interval the ability of the liver to excrete the material is determined. The normal liver does this rapidly, usually removing about 10 to 15 percent per minute. The test is most useful in detecting liver cell damage especially in the absence of jaundice, in cirrhosis, and in chronic hepatitis.

BUN

(See Urea.)

CALCIUM AND PHOSPHORUS

Calcium and phosphorus levels in the blood are in reciprocal relationship and should be considered together. They are both absorbed by the small intestine with the help of vitamin-D and parathyroid hormone and both are excreted in the urine and feces. Most of the calcium and phosphorus after being filtered through the glomerulus is reabsorbed and this is also influenced by parathyroid hormone and vitamin-D.

Calcium is transported in the blood in two forms. Half is unionized protein-bound and the other half is ionized with phosphate. The total concentration is 9-11 mg per 100 ml or 4.5 to 5.5 mEq per liter. The inorganic phosphate level of the plasma is 3-4 mg percent in adults and 4.5 to 6.5 mg in children.

There are many factors involved in the regulation of the concentration of serum calcium and phosphorus. The most important of these is the parathyroid hormone which is secreted when a fall in serum calcium occurs. The hormone causes calcium to be mobilized from the bone by resorption. Calcium absorption from the intestine and the renal tubules is enhanced and phosphate secretion by the renal tubules is increased or its reabsorption by the renal tubules is inhibited. A rise in serum calcium stimulates the secretion of calcitonin from either the thyroid or parathyroid gland, returning the serum calcium to normal. Vitamin-D enhances intestinal absorption of calcium and in its absence serum calcium may decrease with consequent stimulation of the parathyroid gland to raise the calcium level.

The total serum concentration of calcium varies directly with the concentration of serum proteins. The ionized half of calcium varies indirectly with the pH level, decrease in alkalosis or high pH, an increase in acidosis or low pH.

Body deficits of calcium induce compensatory secondary hyperparathyroidism which is difficult to distinguish from primary hyperparathyroidism.

A calcium metabolism disorder may be suspected in a patient with renal calculi, bone disease, convulsions, tetany or even vague complaints of malaise or fatigue.

A 24-hour urine calcium test is important and should be performed after a calcium-free diet for three days. An increased value suggests hyperparathyroidism, a renal tubular acidosis. A decrease may suggest hypothyroidism, hypovitaminosis-D or malabsorption syndrome.

Boeck's sarcoid will show an increase in serum and urine calcium. Serum phosphates are normal and the serum alkaline phosphatase will be increased.

Chronic nephritis will increase the blood phosphate level by decreasing the renal clearance of phosphorus. Serum calcium is decreased because diseased kidneys cannot form the active metabolites of vitamin-D. Because of a drop in calcium level the parathyroid glands become activated, causing bone absorption, then osteoblastic activity which raises the alkaline phosphatase.

Hyperparathyroidism may be due to edema, hyperplasia, or carcinoma. The increased production of parathyroid hormone elevates the serum calcium by accelerating bone resorption and increasing renal tubular and intestinal absorption of calcium. The serum phosphorus level is decreased because of the renal tubular excretion or lack of reabsorption of phosphates. Alkaline phosphatase may be elevated due to osteoblastic activity secondary to bony resorption. The 24-hour urine calcium is elevated.

Hypoparathyroidism with a decrease in production of parathyroid hormone also decreases the renal tubular secretion of phosphate leading to a high serum phosphorus. A low serum calcium is caused by a decrease in intestinal absorption, renal tubular reabsorption and bony resorption of calcium. The alkaline phosphatase is normal and the urine calcium is decreased.

In hypovitaminosis-D the intake of calcium is normal but an insufficient supply of vitamin-D prevents adequate absorption so most is excreted in the feces. The serum calcium should be low but may be normal because of secondary hyperparathyroidism. The serum phosphates are decreased, the alkaline phosphatase is increased, and the urine calcium is decreased.

Malabsorption syndrome, the retention of abnormal amounts of fats in the digestive tract which combine with calcium to form an insoluble soap, causes reduced serum calcium. The phosphate and urine calcium are also decreased and the alkaline phosphatase is increased.

Nephrotic syndrome, cirrhosis of the liver, malnutrition, and other diseases which lower serum protein will lower serum calcium. Secondary hyperparathyroidism usually does because the ionized portion of the calcium is not reduced in concentration.

Renal tubular acidosis presents a picture of acidosis, alkaline urine, high urine calcium and phosphates due to defective renal tubular reabsorption of calcium and phosphates. Secondary hyperparathyroidism may develop, raising the alkaline phosphatase level.

CARBON DIOXIDE

Blood carbon dioxide arises from the oxidation of organic compounds within cells and rapidly diffuses across biological membranes. Carbon dioxide in the lungs diffuses into alveolar air and is expelled. The determination in whole blood, plasma, or serum is of most importance when interpreted with hydrogen-ion concentration in assessing conditions with a disturbance in acid-base balance as in dehydration, renal disease, hypoxia, intoxications, and severe gastroenteric diseases.

It should be reme ,bered that an accurate estimate of pH and CO_2 content cannot be made on samples exposed to air because the CO_2 will escape and the pH will rise.

CATECHOLAMINES

Epinephrine and norepinephrine are B-catechol ethonolamines. Normal urine contains approximately 15% epinephrine and 85% norepinephrine. Norepinephrine is constantly being secreted by sympathetic nerve endings and acts at the site of liberation to maintain vasomotor tone and blood pressure. In emergency it does not give the more general and widespread effect of epinephrine.

Paroxysmal or persistent elevation of catecholamines in the blood or urine is diagnostic of pheochromocytoma or extramedullary chromaffin tumors. Some patients with malignant hypertension also have elevated titres.

CEPHALIN FLOCCULATION

Gamma globulin will flocculate cholesterol emulsified in cephalin. Albumin or an albuminlike molecule is there to inhibit this flocculation. In normal serum no flocculation is present. Hepatic diseases which produce abnormal gamma globulin or reduce the albumin concentration will have a positive cephalin flocculation.

CHOLESTEROL

Cholesterol is synthesized from acetate in the body and is derived from the cholesterol of food stuffs. The concentration of available cholesterol is relatively constant but the serum level rises when the fatty acids of the diet are more saturated. Although most tissues synthesize cholesterol, the liver is the principle site of production. Cholesterol plasma levels are increased by growth hormone, lipid-mobilizing hormone, epinephrine, norepinephrine, cortisol and testosterone; and decreased by ACTH, thyrotropin, insulin, glucogen and estrogen.

Cholesterol levels may be decreased in disease processes such as hyperthyroidism and hepatic disease which may be associated with cholesterol calculi in the biliary tract. Hypercholesterolemia may produce a cholesterol accumulation in atheromatous lesions such as found in arteriosclerosis and atherosclerosis, Schüller-Christian syndrome and xanthomatosis lesions of skin, tendon sheath, and bone. Hypercholesterolemia without the tissue accumulations of cholesterol may be found in hypothyroidism, nephrotic syndromes, hypophysectomy, pancreatitis and diabetes mellitus. Cholesterol has also been noted to stimulate the erythrocyte sedimentation rate.

CREATINE AND CREATININE

Creatine (methylguanidine-acetic acid) and creatinine (the anhydride of creatine) are important in the physiology of muscle contraction. Creatine phosphate is the stored energy source for muscle contraction. The creatine is located intracellularly and is not readily excreted in the urine. The creatinine is a waste product of intracellular creatine and is, therefore, the normally excreted compound.

Observation of creatine in the urine is important in patients with muscle disorders; increased readings are found in myositis, various dystrophies, and myasthenia gravis.

CPK

Creatine (methylguanidine-acetic acid) and creatinine (the production by breaking down phosphocreatine into phosphoric acid and creatine. CPK also acts as the catalyst between adenosine diphosphate (ADP) and adenosine triphosphate (ATP). CPK is found in greatest amounts in skeletal muscle where these reactions occur. Elevated values may be seen in necrosis, trauma, exertion or atrophy of striated muscle, acute myocardial infarction, myocarditis, muscular dystrophy, or acute alcoholic intoxication.

BLOOD ELECTROLYTES

The electrolyte composition of human plasma is composed of cations and anions. The cations are sodium (143), potassium (4.5), calcium (5.0), and magnesium (2.5). These total 155.0 mEq/L of plasma which is the same total for the anions which consist of chloride (104), bicarbonate (29), protein (16), phosphate (2), sulfate (1), and organ acids (3). A complete set of electrolyte readings is rarely ordered; however, the three found in highest concentration are usually done: they consist of sodium (cation), chloride (anion), and bicarbonate (anion). The bicarbonate and chloride anions are totaled and subtracted from the sodium ions. The difference between them usually averages approximately 10 mEq/L in a normal patient. With serious electrolyte imbalance occurring in pathologic processes, the difference may be greater than 10 or less than 5 mEq/L.

	Serum Sodium	Serum Potassium	Serum Bicarbonate	Serum Chloride
Acute Renal Failure	D	I	D	I
Adrenal Cortical Insufficiency	D	I	N or D	D
Chronic Renal Failure	D	N or D	D	N or D
Congestive Heart Failure	N or D	N	N	D
Dehydration	I	N	N or D	I
Diabetic Acidosis	D	N or I or D	D	D
Diabetes Insipidus	N or I	N	D	I
Diarrhea	D	D	D	D
Diuretics:				
Mercurial	D	D	I	D
Chlorothiazide	D	D	D	D
Malabsorption	D	D	N or D	N
Pathologic Diaphoresis	D	N	N	D
Pulmonary Emphysema	I	N	I	D
Pyloric Obstruction	D	D	I	D
Renal Tubular Acidosis	D	D	D	I
Salicylate Toxicity	N	N or D	D	I
Starvation	N	N	D	N

(N = normal; D = decrease; I = increase.)

GLOBULIN

The serum globulins of the blood proteins are usually separated by electrophoresis into the varied globulin fractions. Paper electrophoresis is discussed elsewhere in this text. The globulin fractions are expressed in percentages and include alpha-1 globulin, alpha-2 globulin, beta globulin, and gamma globulin. The alpha and beta globulins may be elevated in liver diseases. Elevated gamma globulins are associated with infectious hepatitis, collagen diseases, carcinomas, and chronic leukemia. They are usually associated with infectious disease since they are antibody fractions.

The serum albumin is seldom elevated and conversely the serum globulins are seldom decreased in disease processes.

The Bence-Jones protein, which is an abnormal globulin is frequently elevated in the blood and excreted in high amounts in the urine in cases of multiple myeloma.

GLUCOSE

Glucose is the main carbohydrate in the body which is stored as glycogen in muscle and liver. When peripheral tissues need glucose, the glycogen converted to glucose is transported by the blood. Glucose is normally filtered through the glomerulus and reabsorbed by the tubule of the kidney, no glucose appearing in the urine. In diabetes mellitus the peripheral tissues lose their ability to take up glucose resulting in an increased blood glucose concentration. The renal tubule is able to absorb only part of the increased blood glucose, and the remainder spills over into the urine.

Blood glucose is regulated directly by two hormones: glucagon, produced in the alpha cells of the islet of Langerhans in the pancreas and insulin, produced in the beta cells. The secretion of glucagon accelerates the breakdown of glycogen in the liver causing an increase in blood glucose. Insulin stimulates the formation of glycogen from glucose in the liver reducing blood glucose levels.

Also contributing to glucose metabolism are ACTH and growth hormone from the pituitary gland, steroids from the adrenal cortex, epinephrine from the adrenal medulla and thyroxine from the thyroid gland.

Hyperglycemia may occur in diabetes mellitus, hyperactivity of adrenals, pituitary, and thyroid glands, sepsis, meningitis, encephalitis, tumors and anoxia.

Hypoglycemia or blood glucose values under 60 mg % occur most frequently in an overdose of insulin and may also be found in myxedema, hypopituitarism, Addison's disease, and glucagon deficiencies.

GLUCOSE TOLERANCE TEST

The patient must have eaten adequate carbohydrates (150 gm a day) for 72 hours prior to testing and should not have been subjected to recent trauma. The patient must be fasting and must be given glucose calculated for his body mass although most are given 100 gm of glucose. The Glucose Tolerance Test will demonstrate the rate of removal of glucose from the bloodstream (Figure 10-4). Factors influencing the curve are the rate at which glucose is absorbed in the gastrointestinal tract and the rate and degree of filtration and reabsorption by the kidney. A flat curve may be caused by a malabsorption syndrome. Low or normal glucose levels with a spillage of glucose in the urine may indicate renal glycosuria. The insulin response to oral glucose in a normal individual is almost immediate, the insulin level peaking between 30 and 60 minutes and returning to normal limits within three hours.

In the diabetic there is little or no secretion of insulin which results in abnormally elevated glucose levels throughout the test.

In maturity-onset diabetes the insulin secretion is delayed and then slightly higher than normal at two hours. The glucose level is therefore elevated until near the two-hour-period.

In the hypoglycemic there is a delay in insulin secretion followed by hypersecretion. The blood glucose is therefore below normal after the two-hour-point until four or five hours because of high insulin levels.

HYDROXYBUTYRIC DEHYDROGENASE (HBD)

Hydroxybutyric Dehydrogenase (HBD) is an enzyme which is found in highest concentration in the heart, skeletal muscle, liver and erythrocytes.

| National Health Laboratories INCORPORATED | 1007 ELECTRIC AVENUE VIENNA, VIRGINIA 22180 PHONE (703) 281-5100 | 10-4 DR. MURRAY POLITZ 121 CONGRESSIONAL LANE ROCKVILLE   MD 20852   RTE L |

PATIENT NAME	SEX	AGE	ACCESSION	DATE OF ACCESSION	DATE OF REPORT	ACCOUNT NO.
DOE JOHN			252201	8/03/77	8-03-77	7081013

TEST	RESULTS	ABNORMAL FLAG	NORMAL VALUES
HEALTH SURVEY VI - (SMA-12)	REPORTED SEPARATELY		
GLUCOSE TOLERANCE - (5 HOUR)			
GLUCOSE -- FASTING	75 MG/DL		65 - 110 FASTING
GLUCOSE TOLERANCE 1/2 HR	115 MG/DL		30 - 60 ABOVE FAST.
GLUCOSE TOLERANCE 1 HR	122 MG/DL		20 - 50 ABOVE FAST.
GLUCOSE TOLERANCE 2 HRS	96 MG/DL		5 - 15 ABOVE FAST.
GLUCOSE TOLERANCE 3 HRS	74 MG/DL		65 - 110
GLUCOSE TOLERANCE 4 HRS	67 MG/DL		65 - 110
GLUCOSE TOLERANCE 5 HRS	71 MG/DL		65 - 110

THIS NEW PERFORATED FORM IS FOR YOUR FILING CONVENIENCE

DAN FERIOZI, M.D. - PATHOLOGIST AND DIRECTOR

FIGURE 10-4: Glucose Tolerance Test. (From National Health Laboratories, Inc., Vienna, Virginia, with permission.)

Tissue damage will cause the HBD and LDH to be elevated. The HBD is more specific than the LDH in myocardial infarction because it may increase up to four times normal value in approximately 48 hours and remains elevated for about 13 days compared to 11 days for the LDH. A polymyositis of several muscle groups may also cause an increase in the HBD.

HIPPURIC ACID (QUICK LIVER FUNCTION TEST)

Some of an ingested quantity of benzoic acid is detoxified in the liver by combination with glycine to form hippuric acid, which is excreted in the urine. The detoxifying power of the liver is diminished in parenchymal liver disease and the rate of hippuric acid excretion in the urine is decreased after a test dose of benzoate. It is important that the patient have normal renal function.

LDH

Serum lactic dehydrogenase are enzymes which act as a catalyst in carbohydrate metabolism. They are active in the pyruvic acid-lactic acid interchange and are found in the kidneys, liver, heart, skeletal muscle and erythrocytes. The LDH is rarely decreased and when increased is not specific. It may be elevated in acute myocardial infarction, congestive heart failure, hepatitis, pernicious anemia, pulmonary embolism infarction, and carcinoma.

17-HYDROXYCORTICOSTEROIDS

17-Hydroxycorticosteroids are steroids produced by the adrenal cortical fasciculata-reticularis. Vital to all facets of metabolism, their main function is to promote homeostatis. In excess, they produce negative nitrogen balance, cessation of growth, muscle wasting, thinning of the skin, osteoporosis and a reduction in lymphoid tissue. If they are insufficient, changes in electrolyte and water metabolism include excessive renal and extra-renal sodium loss, potassium retention, decreased serum sodium, increased serum potassium, metabolic acidosis, decreased intracellular sodium and increased intracellular potassium. There is an increase in the total body water, a decrease in the glomerular filtration rate and inadequate control of blood pressure.

Quantitation of 17-hydroxycorticoids shows they are almost absent in Addison's disease and low in cases of adrenal insufficiency, myxedema, and anterior pituitary insufficiency. There is a marked elevation in Cushing's disease, in moderate thyrotoxicosis, and in stress situations such as those resulting from infectious disease, surgery, or burns. There may be a mild elevation during the first trimester of pregnancy, during severe hypertension and in virilism.

There may also be elevation due to simple obesity since they are correlated with body weight.

ICTERUS INDEX

Icterus index is an expression of the degree of yellow coloration of the blood serum when compared to an artificial standard of potassium dichromate. The test is a simple method for following the degree of jaundice. The ingestion of colored substances such as carotinoids may also cause elevated values.

IRON

Most iron is stored in the form of hemoglobin as myoglobin with the remainder stored in the liver. Iron is present in low concentration in plasma combined with the protein transferrin. The concentration of transferrin limits the iron-binding capacity of the plasma with less than one quarter of the transferrin in combination with iron. Low serum iron is found in acute and chronic diseases, in pregnancy, and in iron-deficiency states usually accompanied by anemia. High values have been seen in hemochromatosis, pernicious anemia and hepatitis.

Serum iron is often determined after the addition of an acid to separate the iron from the protein. If excess iron is then added, the protein becomes saturated with iron. After removal of the excess iron, usually an ion exchange resin, the total iron is determined. The value represents the iron-binding capacity. The iron-binding capacity is decreased in hemochromatosis, the nephrotic syndrome and malignancy.

LIPASE

Lipases are enzymes which catalyze the hydrolysis of long-chain fatty acid esters of glycerol and other polyhydric alcohols. Lipase is produced in the pancreas and secreted into the intestine where it aids in the digestion of fat in the presence of salts. In acute pancreatitis, lipase escapes into the circulation as does amylase. Amylase tends to return to normal within two or three days after the onset of acute pancreatitis, while serum lipase may remain elevated up to two weeks.

LIPIDS

(See **Triglycerides.**)

NON-PROTEIN NITROGEN (NPN)

Non-protein nitrogen (NPN) refers to all nitrogen in biological fluids that is not protein, including amino acids, small peptides, urea, uric acid and creatinine to name a few. The test is usually ordered in cases of suspected renal damage.

TOTAL NITROGEN

Total nitrogen in urine and feces is determined in order to estimate the total excretion of nitrogen from a patient in a 24-hour-period. The nitrogen balance can be calculated from the nitrogen intake and excretion which should be identical when in balance. A larger intake then excretion is termed positive nitrogen balance, while more excretion than intake is called negative nitrogen balance. Increased fecal nitrogen is also indicative of pancreatic function.

PROTEIN BOUND IODINE (PBI)

Ingested inorganic iodide is removed from the circulation and is oxidized to free iodine within the thyroid gland. The iodine combines with tyrosin of the thyroglobulin and is stored in the colloid of the thyroid gland. The colloid also contains mono- and diiodotryosine, triiodothyronine and thryoxine. The pituitary thryoid-stimulating hormone (TSH) causes thyroglobulin to release thyroxine and triiodothyronine into the circulation. Thyroxine is quickly bound to plasma proteins in the blood. One is a glycoprotein called thryoxine-binding globulin (TBG) and the other is thyroxine-binding pre-albumin (TB-

BA). A small amount of thyroxine remains free in the circulation. Iodine is present in the plasma as triiodothyronine (T_3), thyroxine (T_4), and as inorganic iodine which does not relate to thyroid activity.

T_3 is more physiologically active than T_4 but contributes little to the total iodine pool because of its low concentration. Thyroxine contributes most of the protein-bound iodine of the plasma. Thyroxine is so strongly bound to the plasma protein that when the proteins are precipitated, thyroxine precipitates with them and the content of iodine that is precipitated is called the protein-bound iodine (PBI).

There is variation in day-to-day PBI in individuals, related to their metabolic needs and regulated by the amount of thyroxine binding proteins present in their plasma. The PBI is low in cretinism, myxedema, hypothyroidism, acute thyroiditis, and in conditions in which circulating estrogens are abnormally found elevated. An increased PBI may occur in hyperthyroidism, estrogen therapy, pregnancy, early hepatitis, and in patients using birth-control pills.

BLOOD pH

The pH of blood reflects the acid-base balance of the body which is controlled within relatively narrow limits. The mechanism involves production and buffering of acid and its elimination by the body. The measurement has its greatest significance in evaluating the acid-base state of the patient. A pH is indicated anytime a carbon dioxide content is also determined or in any situation in which acidosis or alkalosis is suspected. Venous blood 7.36—7.40; arterial 7.38—7.42.

PHOSPHATASE: ALKALINE AND ACID

The phosphatases are a group of enzymes found in the body and are categorized on the basis of the pH at which they exhibit maximum activity. The alkaline phosphatases are maximally active at a pH of 9—10 and are distributed widely in the body. They are important in digestion and mucosal absorption since they are necessary for hydrolysis of organic phosphates. Osteoblastic activity is also associated with increased alkaline phosphatase.

Acid phosphatase levels of 0.2—0.8 Bodansky units or 1—4 King-Armstrong units per 100 ml are normal. This test is most useful in the diagnosis of carcinoma of the prostate, although it may also be elevated in Gaucher's disease and in hemopoietic disturbances.

Alkaline phosphatase levels of 1—4 Bodansky units or 8—14 King-Armstrong units per 100 ml are normal. In growth and development years normal values may be 5—15 Bodansky units due to increased osteoblastic activity. General debility and anemia are associated with lower values. This test is very useful in differentiation of various bone diseases and hyperparathyroidism when combined with tests for serum calcium and phosphorus.

The alkaline phosphatase is usually elevated in obstructive jaundice and rarely elevated in hepatocellular jaundice.

The relationship of the phosphatases to different bone diseases are presented below.

METASTATIC BONE TUMORS
Metastatic and primary bone neoplasms may produce osteoblastic activity and thus lead to an elevated alkaline phosphatase. If the metastases are from the prostate gland, an elevated acid phosphatase may also be present.

Osteoblastic metatases may be associated with carcinoma of the breast, kidney, or thyroid, and Hodgkin's disease. Metastatic carcinomas which may produce osteolytic lesions with no rise in alkaline phosphatase levels are from the lungs, rectum, kidney, and breasts.

OSTEITIS DEFORMANS (PAGET'S DISEASE)
This disease is characterized by an idiopathic localized bone destruction and reabsorption, followed by compensatory abnormal new bone formation as depicted in radiologic studies of the skull and long bones. The alkaline phosphatase may reach its highest levels of 100 or more Bodansky units.

PRIMARY BONE TUMORS
Osteoblastic bone tumors such as osteogenic sarcoma, chondrosarcoma and malignant giant-cell tumor are associated with an increased alkaline phosphatase of 20 to 40 times normal.

Osteolytic lesions associated with bone tumors such as osteogenic sarcoma do not affect the alkaline phosphatase.

Serum calcium and phosphorus levels are normal; in massive invasions, however, the calcium level may rise and steroids are needed to bring it down.

RICKETS AND OSTEOMALACIA

Rickets and osteomalacia have low blood calcium causing an increase in parathyroid activity which induces reabsorption of bone to compensate for the low blood calcium. The bone reacts with increased osteoblastic activity and raises the alkaline phosphatase. Primary hyperparathyroidism also produces the same picture. Whenever a low blood calcium level occurs from either inadequate intake or absorption or increased urinary excretion, a rise in alkaline phosphatase occurs.

PHOSPHORUS

(See **Calcium**.)

POTASSIUM

Potassium is the major cation of intracellular fluid. The concentration of potassium in extracellular fluid is much less with sodium being the main cation. The cell membrane maintains the concentration gradients between sodium and potassium which is important in membrane potentials in muscles. Alteration of the gradient alters the excitability of the membranes.

Serum potassium increases in adrenal cortical insufficiency, renal failure, anuria, dehydration, and cellular breakdown.

Serum potassium decreases result from decreased intake, loss from the alimentary tract, or increased excretion by the kidneys. Decreased serum potassium is also demonstrated in vomiting, diarrhea, and in Cushing's syndrome.

TOTAL PLASMA PROTEIN

Protein is found in all body fluids as mixtures which may be separated into its numerous components by several means such as differential precipitation, ultra-centrifugation, immunochemical techniques, and electrophoresis. The body fluid proteins, especially those of the plasma, are concerned with nutrition, water distribution, acid-base balance, transport mechanism, coagulation, immunity, and enzymatic action.

Proteins possess a common basic chemical constitution but diversify enormously in size and function.

Total plasma protein concentration as well as alteration in the relative concentration of the major components occur in a great many diseases and are of clinical value; however, they are not definitive diagnostically. The total protein tends to decrease in abnormal conditions. The decrease is usually in the concentration of albumin; however, the globulin will usually increase. Although the reciprocal changes in albumin may result in a normal protein, it is usually below normal.

PROTEIN ELECTROPHORESIS

The measurement of colloidal particles in an electronic field is called electrophoresis. The intensity of the electrical field along with particle size and shape and electrical charge are important factors.

Serum proteins are most commonly subjected to electrophoresis for identification and quantitation. In the electrical field different proteins migrate at different rates because they are different in electric charge, size, and shape.

Sunderman and Sunderman have listed pathologic conditions in which electrophoretic patterns of serum are specifically altered from the normal, including hepatic cirrhosis, viral hepatitis, nephrosis, scleroderma, lupus erythematosus, rheumatoid arthritis, Boeck's sarcoid, multiple myeloma, lymphatic leukemia, lymphomas, myelogenous leukemia, monocytic leukemia, Hodgkin's disease, and hypogammaglobulinemia. Jencks and associates also include tuberculosis, malignant neoplasms, arteriosclerosis, rheumatoid heart disease, sarcoidosis, kala-azar and lymphogranuloma venereum.

SODIUM

Sodium is the major cation of extracellular fluid with a very low concentration intercellularly. The concentration differences are important in maintaining the electrical membrane potentials of muscle. Serum sodium levels decrease in the vomiting and diarrhea which are common to uremia, diabetic coma, toxemia, pyloric stenosis, ulcerative colitis, and infections of the alimentary tract. Serum sodium levels increase in dehydration, renal failure, and cardiac failure.

SULPHENOGLOBIN

Sulphenoglobin is an altered form of hemoglobin. It may be formed in the body by the action of certain drugs such as phenacetin, the sulfonamides, and Bromo Seltzer®°; many of these also cause methemoglobinemia. Sulphenoglobin may be present alone or in conjunction with methemoglobin. Sulphenoglobin interferes with the ability of hemoglobin to carry oxygen. Arterial and capillary blood take on a brownish hue if the concentration of sulphenoglobin becomes sufficiently high.

THYMOL TURBIDITY

Thymol turbidity is a test which measures the degree of turbidity produced when serum is mixed with a buffered solution of thymol. Minimal turbidity occurs in normal serum; greater turbidity is seen in certain conditions, especially parenchymatous liver disease. Increased results are also seen in infectious hepatitis, cirrhosis, Weil's disease and metastatic neoplasm of the liver. Lipemic serum may give a false positive and cause a nonspecific increase in turbidity.

TRANSAMINASES

Transaminases are enzymes which catalyze the transfer of amino groups from an amino acid to a keto acid. They show a fairly high degree of specificity and are named for the amino acid and keto acid substances on which they act. Glutamic-oxalacetic transaminase (GOT) and glutamic-pyruvic transaminase (GPT) have gained clinical importance. The GOT is particularly high in the heart and liver and the GPT is most active in the liver. Damage to these tissues results in an increase in the serum level of the enzymes. The SGOT is useful in the diagnosis of myocardial infarction and in the early detection of liver damage. It is also elevated in muscular dystrophy and renal infarction but not pulmonary infarction. The SGPT is more

°Bristol-Myers, Syracuse, New York

specific than GOT for liver cell necrosis; both are widely used in diagnosis. Drugs which affect the SGOT and LDH are opiates and oral contraceptives.

TRANSAMINASE CHART

	Transaminase	Lactic Dehydrogenase	CPK
Cardiac Failure	Increased	Normal or increased	Normal
Dermotomyositis	Increased	Increased	Increase
Extraphepatic Biliary Obstruction	Increased	Normal	Normal
Myocardial Infarction	Increased	Increased	Normal
Pulmonary Infarction	Normal	Increased	Normal
Viral Hepatitis	Increased	Normal or increased	Normal

T_3 T_4 T_7

T_3 UPTAKE

The uptake of triiodothyronine by red blood cells is a method of estimating thyroid function. Because it is a test *in vitro*, the procedure avoids the administration of radioactive materials to the patient, and does not require the patient's presence or cooperation for completion of the test. The test also permits the evaluation of thyroid function under circumstances where other thyroid function tests are not valid because of previous iodine medication for diagnostic or therapeutic purposes. The test is a measure of the binding power of the plasma proteins for L-triiodothyronine and is not a measure of metabolism of the erythrocytes. In hyperthyroidism there is an increase in circulating thyroid hormone to occupy the binding sites of the plasma proteins. The T_3 uptake may be elevated in hyperthyroidism, severe nephrosis, prolonged iodine deficiency, pregnancy, and carcinoma.Certain drugs will also cause an elevation, including hormones, steroids, penicillin, and Butazolidin®° with salicylates or Dilantin®°°. The T₃ uptake may be normal in nontoxic goiter or thyroid carcinoma. T₃ may be decreased in hypothyroidism, panhypopituitarism or Simmond's disease and after iodine or antithyroid preparation and with birth-control pills.

T₄ TESTS

The T₄ may be a more reliable test for thyroid studies because the T₃ is affected by outside factors including drugs and estrogens. T₄ normal is 3.4–11.2 mg/ml.

T₇ TESTS

The T₇, which is fairly new, is based on the T₃ and T₄ and is arrived at by the formula:

$$\frac{T_3}{100} \ \text{x} \ \ T_4 \ = \ T_7$$

The T₇ normal range is 0.85–3.92 mg/ml.

TRIGLYCERIDES

Triglycerides are the blood lipids or fat and are esters of glycerol and fatty acids. The triglycerides along with cholesterol and phospholipids form the main blood lipids.

Triglycerides along with glucose and inorganic phosphorus are altered by dietary intake; the tests should be run after a fast.

Triglycerides are increased in hypothyroidism and several familial enzyme-deficiency abnormalities. A lipoprotein electrophoresis is used to separate the five distinct types of familial hyperlipemia conditions with serum triglycerides, phospholipids, and PBI to exclude hyper- and hypothyroidism.

UREA

Urea is formed in the liver from groups of amino acids and is the end product of nitrogen metabolism. The urea is excreted by the

°GEIGY Pharmaceuticals, Ardsley, New York
°°Parke, Davis & Co., Detroit, Michigan

kidneys. Hepatic disease may diminish the ability of the liver to form urea, resulting in low levels of urea and high levels of ammonia in the blood. Renal failure results in the inability to excrete urea, thus increasing the blood urea concentration. Values slightly higher than normal are found in the elderly, and lower in persons on inadequate diets. Decreases in the urea levels are rare. Higher values are found in diarrhea, diabetic coma, Addison's disease, shock following burns, cardiac failure, glomerulonephritis, nephrosis, renal calculi, lower-urinary-tract obstruction, and where there is reduced volume of body fluid from vomiting due to intestinal obstruction.

URIC ACID

Uric acid is the metabolic end product of purines. In gout the pool of uric acid is increased and urates are deposited in and around joints, producing the characteristic pain and swelling. In gout or gouty arthritis the uric acid level is increased and usually suspected. Renal failure can result in an increase in blood uric acid and should be ruled out. Increases in the uric acid level are also found in toxemia of pregnancy, leukemia, pneumonia, polycythemia, multiple myeloma, lymphoblastomas, chronic glomerulonephritis; these increases, however, are not diagnostically as important as in gout.

VANILLYLMANDELIC ACID (VMA)

Vanillylmandelic acid (VMA) is the urinary metabolite of both epinephrine and norephinephine and therefore reflects the endogenous secretions of catecholamines. It is usually wise to measure both catecholamines and vanillylmandelic acid (VMA) because one may be elevated and the other not. The measurement of urinary VMA rather than of catecholamines has gained favor because of the relatively large quantities of urinary UMA in the urine as compared to the catecholamines.

CHAPTER 11

Diagnostic Test Procedures

BASIC SCREENING—12 TESTS (SMA-12)*

Calcium	Albumin
Phosphorus	Total protein
Glucose	Alk. phosphatase
BUN	SGOT
Bilirubin, total	LDH
Cholesterol	Uric acid

*See Figure 11-1.

ANEMIA

CBC with differential and indices
Platelet count
Reticulocyte count

ATHEROSCLEROSIS

Glucose	Total lipids
Cholesterol	Triglycerides

CLOTTING TESTS

Bleeding time (platelets and integrity of vessel wall)
Partial thromboplastin (Stage I), intrinsic
Prothrombin time (Stage II), extrinsic

TESTS FOR EDEMA

CBC	Addis count
Urine	PBI
Sedimentation rate	Renal function test
Na, L, Cl, CO_2	24-Hour Urine—17-Ketosteroids
Serum protein and A/G ratio	and 17-Hydroxysteroids

189

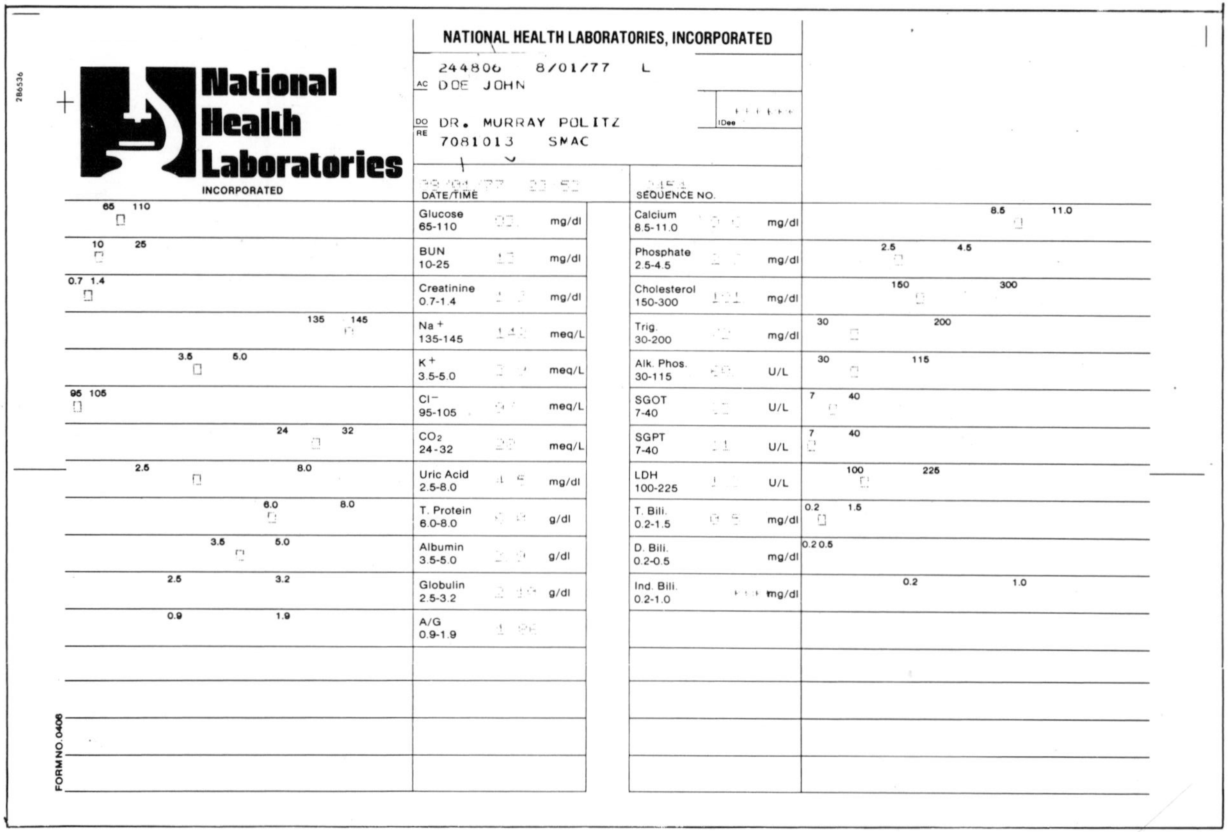

FIGURE 11-1: Basic screening tests. (From National Health Laboratories, Inc., Vienna, Virginia, with permission.)

HEMATOLOGIC DISEASE—CHEMISTRIES

Iron   LDH
Total bilirubin

HYPERTENSION

Urinary VMA   Cholesterol
Catecholamines   Triglycerides
BUN

JOINT-PAIN OR SWELLING

Most Often Ordered:
  CBC
  Sedimentation rate
  ASO titre
  CRP
  RA test
  Sickle-cell prep.
  LE prep and ANA
  Uric acid

Less Frequently Ordered:
  Febrile agglutinin
  Heterophile antibody titer
  Eosinophil count (trichnosis, periarteritis)
  Synovial analysis
  Synovial culture (bacteria, fungi, spirochetes)
  Coagulation time (hemophilia)
  Serum protein electrophoresis

LIVER DISEASE

Total protein   SGO-transaminase
Albumin   SGP-transaminase
A/G ratio   LDH
Total bilirubin   G-glutamyl transpep
Globulin   Alkaline phosphatase
Direct bilirubin

MYOCARDIAL INFARCTION

SGO-transaminase	LDH (lactic dehydrogenase)

PANCREATITIS

Amylase

PARATHYROID DISEASE

Calcium	BUN
Phosphorus	Alkaline phosphatase

PREOPERATIVE TESTS FOR BONE SURGERY (MINIMAL)*

CBC with differential and indices	Uric acid
	P.T.
Sedimentation rate	P.T.T.
Glucose	Urinalysis

*See Figure 11-2.

PURPURA

CBC	Rumple-Leede test
Sedimentation rate	Thromboplastin generation test
Coagulation time and P.T.T.	L.E. and ANA
Bleeding time	Heterophile antibody titre
Prothrombin time	Cold agglutinins
Platelet count	

RENAL DISEASE

BUN	Albumin
Creatinine	Sodium
BUN/creatinine ratio	Potassium
Total protein	Chloride
Globulin	A/G ratio

THYROID DISEASE

PBI	Cholesterol
T_3, T_4, T_7	Serum TSH (Thyroid
Free thryoxine	Stimulating Hormone)

National Health Laboratories INCORPORATED

1007 ELECTRIC AVENUE
VIENNA, VIRGINIA 22180
PHONE (703) 281-5100

DR. MURRAY POLITZ

PATIENT NAME	SEX	AGE	ACCESSION	DATE OF ACCESSION	DATE OF REPORT	ACCOUNT NO.
DOE JOHN			244787	8/01/77	8-01-77	7081013

TEST	RESULTS	ABNORMAL FLAG	NORMAL VALUES
PODIATRIST PRE-OPERATIVE GROUP			
COMPLETE BLOOD COUNT			
HEMATOCRIT	32.5 VOL%		M: 42-52 - F: 37-47
HEMOGLOBIN	10.4 G/DL		M: 14-18 - F: 12-16
RED BLOOD COUNT	4.71 MILLION /CU.MM		MALE: 4.7 - 6.0
			FEMALE: 4.0 - 5.4
WHITE BLOOD COUNT	5.3 THOUS/CU.MM.		5 - 11
LYMPH	34 %		20 - 40
SEG	65 %		50 - 70
MONO	1 %		1 - 6
% ATL	00 %		
HYPOCHROMIA	1+		
ANISOCYTOSIS	2+		
POIKILOCYTOSIS	2+		
M C V	69 CU. MICRONS		M: 80-94 - F: 81-99
M C H	22.0 MICRO-MICRO GM		27 - 31
M C H C	32.0 %		32 - 36
COMMENTS:	ADEQUATE PLATELETS ***		MALE: 0 - 10
SEDIMENTATION RATE-WINTROBE	11 MM/HR		FEMALE: 0 - 20
PROTHROMBIN TIME			
CONTROL - PT	12 SECONDS		
PATIENT - PT	13 SECONDS		
% ACTIVITY	89 %		
PARTIAL THROMBOPLASTIN TIME			
CONTROL - PTT	32 SECONDS		35 - 45
PATIENT - PTT	35 SECONDS		35 - 45
GLUCOSE, PLASMA	102 MG/DL		65 - 110 (FASTING)
URIC ACID - SERUM	3.9 MG/DL		M: 2 - 8 * F: 2 - 6
URINALYSIS - ROUTINE			
COLOR	YELLOW		
APPEARANCE	CLEAR		
REACTION	ACID		
SPECIFIC GRAVITY	1.022		
GLUCOSE	NEG		
ALBUMIN	NEG		
ACETONE	NEG		
WBC/HPF	0-2		
RBC/HPF	NONE SEEN		
EPITH CELLS	0-1		
BACTERIA	NONE SEEN		
CRYSTALS	NONE SEEN		
CASTS	NONE SEEN		

*** CBC TEST RAN TWICE

2+ MICROCYTES

CORRECTED COPY

THIS NEW PERFORATED FORM IS FOR YOUR FILING CONVENIENCE

DAN FERIOZI, M.D. - PATHOLOGIST AND DIRECTOR

FIGURE 11-2: Preoperative Blood and Urine Test showing anemia. (From National Health Laboratories, Inc., Vienna, Virginia, with permission.)

Bibliography

Abel, R. et al in consultation: Which lab tests for which patient? *Patient Care*, **6**: 41, June, 1972.

Addino, J.G.: Hyperlipidemia and tendinous xanthoma. *J. Foot Surg.*, **13**: 1, 1974.

Alexander, J.W.: Host defense mechanism against infection. *Surg. Clin. N. Am.*, **52**: 1367, December, 1972.

Annino, T.S. and Relman, A.S.: The effect of eating on some of the clinically important chemical constituents of blood. *Am. J. Clin. Pathol.*, **31**: 155, 1959.

Bauer, J.D. et al: *Clinical Laboratory Methods*, 8th edition, C.V. Mosby Co., St. Louis, 1974.

Bauer, J.D. et al: *Clinical Laboratory Methods*, 7th edition, C.V. Mosby Co., St. Louis, 1974.

Beeson, P.B. and McDermott, W. (Editors): *Textbook of Medicine*, 11th edition, W.B. Saunders Co., 1963.

Blumberg, R.S., Bunim, J.T., Elkins, E., Pironi, C.L., and Zvaifler, N.J.: ARA nomenclature and classification of arthritis and rheumatism (tentative). *Arthritis Rheum.*, **7**: 93, 1964.

Bomford, R.R. et al: *Hutchinson's Clinical Methods*, 14th edition, Lippincott, Philadelphia, 1963.

Boyd, W.: *A Textbook of Pathology*, 7th edition, Lea and Febiger, Philadelphia, 1961.

Carrel, J.L., Carrel, J.M., and Davidson, D.M.: Lipid disorders in podiatric practice—atypical gout? *JAPA*, **60**: 448, 1970.

Carrel, J.L., Carrel, J.M., Davidson, D.M.: Differential diagnosis of acute arthralgias of the foot. *JAPA*, **61**: 256, 1971.

Carrel, J.L., Carrel, J.M., and Davidson, D.M.: Pitfalls in the evaluation of clinical laboratory results. *J. Foot Surg.*, **11**: 2, 1972.

Carrel, J.M. and Davidson, D.M.: Current concepts of coagulation and their application to podiatric surgery. *JAPA*, **65**: 1, January, 1975.

Cartledge, W.: Hemostasis in digital surgery. *JAPA*, **6**: 6, pp. 423–426, June, 1962.

Collins, R.D.: *Illustrated Manual of Laboratory Diagnosis*, 2nd edition, Lippincott, Philadelphia, 1975.

Committee on Pre- and Postoperative Care of the American College of Foot Surgeons: *Manual of Preoperative and Postoperative Care*, W.B. Saunders Co., Philadelphia, 1967.

Curin, G., Peters, W.J., and Tsoutsooris, G.V.: A study of infections in the foot. *JAPA*, **65**: 7, July, 1975.

Damm, H.C. and King, J.W.: *Handbook of Clinical Laboratory Data*, The Chemical Rubber Co., Cleveland, 1965.

Davidsohn, I. and Henry, J.B. (Editors): *Todd-Sanford Clinical Diagnosis by Laboratory Methods*, 15th edition, W.B. Saunders Co., 1974.

Davidson, S.S.: *The Principles and Practice of Medicine*, Williams and Wilkins Co., Baltimore, 1968.

Davison, S.: Local manifestations in the lower extremities of systemic diseases. *JAPA*, **48**: 7, pp. 294–303, July, 1958.

Dorland's Illustrated Medical Dictionary, 24th edition, W.B. Saunders Co., Philadelphia, 1965.

Duvrie, H.L.: *Surgery of the Foot*, 5th edition, V.T. Inman (Editor), C.V. Mosby Co., St. Louis, 1973.

Frankel, S. et al: *Graduhol's Clinical Laboratory Methods and Diagnosis: A Textbook on Laboratory Procedures and Their Interpretation*, 7th edition, C.V. Mosby Co., 1970.

Frobisher, M.: *Fundamentals of Microbiology*, W.B. Saunders Co., Philadelphia, 1965.

Giannestras, N.: *Foot Disorders*, Lea and Febiger, Philadelphia, 1967.

Goodman, L.S. and Gilman. A.: *The Pharmaceutical Basis of Therapeutics*, 4th edition, MacMillan, New York, 1970.

Greenbury, C.L.: A comparison of the Rose-Waculaer, latex-fixation, Ra test, and bentonite flocculation tests. *Am. J. Clin. Pathol.*, **13**: 4, July, 1960.

Hara, B. et al: *Complications in Foot Surgery*, Williams and Wilkins Co., Baltimore, 1976.

Harrison, T.R.: *Harrison's Principles of Internal Medicine*, McGraw Hill, New York, 1974.

Hilleboe, H.B. and Larimore, G.W.: *Preventative Medicine*, W.B. Saunders Co., Philadelphia, 1965.

Hollander, S.L.: *Arthritis and Allied Conditions*, 7th edition, Lea and Febiger, Philadelphia, 1966.

Jencks, W.P., Smith, E.R.B., and Durrum, E.L.: The clinical significance of the analysis of serum protein distribution by filter paper electrophoresis. *Am. J. Med.*, 21: 387, 1956.

Kalish, S.R. and Irwin, W.G.: Hyperthyroidism-ostteoporosis: A case study in differential diagnosis. *JAPA*, 64: 1, January, 1974.

Kaplan, G.S.: Postoperative infections of the foot. *J. Foot Surg.*, 11: 2 (summer volume), 1972.

Klemperer, P.: The concept of collagen disease in medicine. *Amer. Rev. Resp. Dis.*, 83: 331, 1961.

Levine, M.E. and O'Neal, L.W.: *The Diabetic Foot*, C.V. Mosby Co., St. Louis, 1973.

Marsden, P. and McKerren, G.G.: Serum triodothyronine concentration in the diagnosis of hyperthyroidism. *Clin. Endocrinol.*, 4: 183–185, 1975.

Marsden, P. et al: Hormonal patterns of relapse in hyperthyroidism. *Lancet*, pp. 944–947, April 26, 1975.

Mason, M. and Currey, H.L.: *Clinical Rheumatology*, Lippincott, Philadelphia, 1970.

Medical Services Company of Arizona: *Quick Reference Laboratory Manual for the Physician*, 1973.

Minnefor, A., Olson, M., and Carver, D.: Pseudomonas osteoteomyelitis following puncture wounds of the foot. *J. Foot Surg.*, vol. 11, November 3, 1972.

Nott, D.: Pitfalls in surgery of the foot: Gout. *J. Foot Surg.*, 11: 2, 1972.

O'Keefe, K.: Confessions of a reformed E.R. order writer. *MLO/M. Lab. Observer*, 5: 41, Fall, 1973.

Pack, L.: Burning feet: A partial guide to diagnosis. *Arch. of Pod. Med. Foot Surg.*, 11: 1, July, 1974.

Pack, L.: Acute adult inflammatory pedal arthritis: A practical guide to diagnosis. *JAPA*, 66: 9, 1976.

Parker, R.H. and Paterson, P.Y.: Antimicrobial agents selection and use. *J. Chronic Dis.*, 21: 719, April, 1969.

Price, E.C.: Hematology and urinalysis for chiropody. *J. Nat. Assoc. Chirop.*, 45: 8, 1955.

Pukaski, E.J.: *Common Bacterial Infections—Pathophysiology and Clinical Management*, W.B. Saunders Co., Philadelphia, 1964.

Rebell, G., Taplin, D., and Blank, H.: *Dermatohytes: Their Recognition and Identification*, Dermatology Foundation of Miami, 1964.

Rogovin, J.M.: Basic concepts of postoperative infections. *J. Foot Surg.*, **11**: 2, 1972.

Rosenthal, S.: Mycology in podiatric practice and interpretation of results. In *Podiatric Cross Section*, Westwood Pharmaceuticals, **2**: 1.

Rosenthal, S.A., Fine, H.L., and Baer, R.L.: Present day incidence of superficially infecting pathogenic fungi. *Arch. Dermatol.*, **96**: 15, 1967.

Roven, M.D.: Investigation and identification and treatment of onychomycosis. *Curr. Podiatry*, **25**: 5, May, 1976.

Rubin, L.: The latex fixation test—an office procedure for the detection of rheumatoid arthritis in podiatric patients. *JAPA*, **54**: 11, pp. 771—775, November, 1964.

Salasa, R.M. et al: Postoperative adrenal cortical insufficiency occurrences in patients previously treated with cortisone. *JAMA*, **152**: 16, p. 1509, 1953.

Senrad, A.M.: *Comprehensive Review for Medical Technologists*, C.V. Mosby Co., St. Louis, 1975.

Shalet, S.M., Beardswell, C.G., and Lamb, A.M.: Value of routine serum triiodothyronine estimation in diagnosis of thyrotoxisosis. *Lancet*, pp. 1008—1010, November, 1975.

Shapiro, S.L.: Standardized admitting and nursing orders for in-hospital surgical patients. *J. Foot Surg.*, **11**: 3, 1972.

Shecter, G.O. and Gibson, A.A.: Laboratory tests in chiropody. *J. Nat. Assoc. Chirop.*, **42**: 1, pp. 43—45, January, 1952.

Simon, S.J.S. and Gentzkow, G.J.: *Medical and Public Health Lab Methods*, Lea and Febiger, Philadelphia, 1956, pp. 82—87.

Sirridge, M.: *Laboratory Diagnosis of Haemostasis*, Lea and Febiger, Philadelphia, 1967.

Streiker, F.B.: Foot ulcers resulting from polycythemia vera. *J. Nat. Assoc. Chirop.*, **45**: 7, July, 1955.

Sunderman, F.U., Jr., and Sunderman, F.W.: Clinical applications of the fractionation of serum proteins by paper electrophoresis. *Am. J. Clin. Path.*, **27**: 125, 1957.

Swater, F.E.: *Textbook of Microbiology*, C.V. Mosby Co., St. Louis, 1967.

Taplin, D., Saias, N., Rebel, G., and Blank, H.: Isolation and recognition of dermatophytes on a new medium (DTM). *Arch. of Dermatol.*, **99**: 203, 1969.

Wallach, J.: *Interpretations of Diagnostic Tests*, Little, Brown and Co., Boston, 1970.

Weinstein, F.: *Principles and Practice of Podiatry*, Lea and Febiger, Philadelphia, 1968.

White, W.L. et al: *Chemistry for Medical Technologists*, 3rd edition, C.V. Mosby Co., St. Louis, 1971.

Widman, F.K.: *Goodale's Clinical Interpretation of Laboratory Tests*, 7th edition, F.A. Davis Co., Philadelphia, 1973.

William, R.H.: *Textbook of Endocrinology*, W.B. Saunders Co., Philadelphia, 1968.

Woolf, W.H.: Verrucae: Its possible relationship to other neoplasms. *JAPA*, **52**: 11, pp. 893−898, November, 1962.

Wyle, W.D. and Churchill-Davidson, H.C.: *A Practice of Anesthesia*, 2nd edition, Yearbook Medical Publishers, Chicago, 1966.

Yale, I.: *Podiatric Medicine*, Williams and Wilkins Co., Baltimore, 1974.

INDEX